12

Effective
Ways to
Help Your
ADD/ADHD
Child

LAURA J. STEVENS, M.S.

AVERY
a member of
Penguin Putnam Inc.
New York

12

Effective Ways to Help Your ADD/ADHD Child

Drug-Free Alternatives for Attention-Deficit Disorders

Most Avery books are available at special quantity discounts for bulk purchase for sales promotions, premiums, fund-raising, and educational needs. Special books or book excerpts also can be created to fit specific needs. For details, write Putnam Special Markets, 375 Hudson Street, New York, NY 10014.

Avery
a member of
Penguin Putnam Inc.
375 Hudson Street
New York, NY 10014
www.penguinputnam.com

Library of Congress Cataloging-in-Publication Data

Stevens, Laura J., date.
12 effective ways to help your ADD/ADHD child:
drug-free alternatives for attention-deficit disorders / Laura J. Stevens.
p. cm.
Includes index.
ISBN 1-58333-039-9
1. Attention-deficit hyperactivity disorder.   2. Attention-deficit hyperactivity disorder—
Alternative treatment.   3. Attention-deficit hyperactivity disorder—Diet therapy.
1. Title: Twelve effective ways to help your ADD/ADHD child.   II. Title.
RJ506.H9 S718   2000   00-038095
618.92'858906—dc21

Printed in the United States of America
10 9 8 7 6 5 4 3 2 1

To George, my best friend, with all my love

CONTENTS

ACKNOWLEDGMENTS

I thank the following people who have taught and guided me for many years: Dorothy Boyce, R.N., John O'Brian, M.D., Sidney M. Baker, M.D., and Leo Galland, M.D. I admire their dedication and efforts to help children and adults who suffer from behavior, learning, and health problems. I also thank William G. Crook, M.D., for his friendship and enthusiasm for this book. He has taught me much of what I know about food sensitivities and other factors that influence behavior and health. I must thank, too, John R. Burgess, Ph.D., who has guided me in graduate school and beyond and has always insisted upon excellence in research.

I am grateful to Rudy Shur, Elaine Sparber, Dara Stewart, and John Duff at Avery and Penguin Putnam, and appreciate their efforts to shape this book and make it reader-friendly.

Finally, I thank my family for their love and support.

FOREWORD

If your child has been diagnosed with ADD or ADHD, you'll find Laura Stevens's new book invaluable, since it contains information you cannot find elsewhere. It's comprehensive, yet concise. It's well organized and user-friendly.

Who is Laura J. Stevens, and why am I so enthusiastic about her book? Here are only a few of the reasons: I've known Laura for more than fifteen years. Together, we wrote a 1987 book, *Solving the Puzzle of Your Hard-to-Raise Child.*

Laura wrote other books in the early 1980s dealing with children now labeled as having ADD or ADHD. At that time, these children were called hyperactive, allergic, lazy, and/or irritable. And Laura provided parents and professionals with answers.

Also, because of her generous and warm personality, Laura has helped thousands of parents whose children were troubled by behavior and learning problems. She's done a little of this in person, and a lot more through her web page on the Internet.

Here's more: Laura is a mother and a highly educated professional. She is now carrying out research (in collaboration with colleagues at Purdue University) on the critically important role of the good fats (the omega-3 fatty acids) in helping children with behavior, learning, and other health problems.

As Laura points out in the introduction to this book, helping the child with ADD or ADHD is like solving a jigsaw puzzle. You have to identify the biological and nutritional pieces, and then fit them together into a completed puzzle. Although this task may seem daunting, it is more important for you to accomplish it now than it was a few years ago. Why? Because scientific studies show that sensitivities to common dietary ingredients play a major role in causing ADHD.

Your physician may have heard about the November 1999 conference sponsored by Georgetown University and the International Health Foundation—ADHD: Causes and Possible Solutions. Participants included pediatricians and other health-care professionals from Yale, MIT, the University of Texas and University of California, and other schools, along with parents and teachers. In their presentations, these professionals discussed the role of nutritionally deficient diets, food allergies and sensitivities, environmental toxins, the repeated use of antibiotics, and yeast overgrowth. Their conclusions: All these factors play an important role in causing behavior and learning problems in children.

Laura's book provides you with a step-by-step approach to putting together the pieces of your child's puzzle. Laura also encourages working with your physician, your child's teacher, and other professionals who have been trying to help.

In addition, Laura discusses Ritalin, and she acknowledges that stimulant medicines may *temporarily* help control the symptoms of ADHD. But if you're like many parents, you're concerned about keeping your child on Ritalin. Here's why: *Ritalin does not provide long-term improvement in academic achievement or a reduction in the possibility of antisocial behavior or arrest rate.*

A final reason why I like this book shows a part of my bias. One of the twelve ways Laura includes in her book is solving the yeast connection. As you may know, I'm certain that yeast plays an important role in causing problems in children ranging from ADD and ADHD to chronic fatigue syndrome and autism.

A final word: Read this book. In my opinion, it will be the best-selling book for parents in the first decade of the twenty-first century.

William G. Crook, M.D.
Emeritus Fellow, American Academy of Pediatrics
Author of *The Yeast Connection Handbook*

PREFACE

If your child is inattentive and impulsive, your doctor may have told you that he has attention-deficit disorder (ADD). If he is also restless, unable to sit still, and overactive, your doctor may have labeled him as having attention-deficit hyperactivity disorder (ADHD). If you are frustrated, confused, and exhausted, you have a lot of company. More than 2 million children in the United States are thought to have ADD or ADHD.

Helping your child with behavior and health problems resembles solving a jigsaw puzzle. Different children have different puzzle pieces. For example, for one child, one "piece" of the puzzle might be sensitivities to common foods and additives. A "piece" for another child might be a marginal iron deficiency. You and your doctor will have to identify the nutritional and biochemical "pieces" of the puzzle that are important for *your* child and fit them together to form a completed puzzle of a healthy, happy, emotionally stable child.

Twenty-five years ago, Linda struggled to help her two hyperactive sons.

She was amazed at how much they improved when she made simple dietary changes. They almost became different children. I've been following Linda's story for many years. Her children's problems were severe and complicated, and help illustrate how to identify the various pieces of the puzzle. As Linda tells the story:

My husband and I were so excited when our first son, Tommy, was born. But Tommy screamed with colic for nine long months. As he learned to sit up, crawl, and walk, he was in constant motion, either rocking back and forth or jumping up and down. Simple tasks frustrated him, and he cried easily and often. Yet many times he smiled and laughed. We felt like failures as parents.

When Tommy was three, my husband and I consulted a clinical child psychologist at the university who recommended that we use M&M's candies to reward good behavior. Tommy's behavior deteriorated so rapidly that we wondered whether the M&M's might be responsible. Reports that diet might affect behavior were just starting to appear in newspapers and magazines.

When Tommy was four, we consulted a pediatric neurologist at a major medical center, who concluded that Tommy was hyperactive [the term "attention-deficit hyperactivity disorder" had not yet been coined], and would probably experience severe learning problems in school and always require special-education classes. A trial of the stimulant drug Ritalin didn't help. In fact, it turned Tommy into a zombie.

When we asked the pediatric neurologist about diet and hyperactivity, he replied, "Oh, there's no relationship. That's just a fad." But we were so desperate, we decided to try the Feingold Diet [popularized by pediatric allergist Benjamin Feingold in the 1970s]. This diet excludes artificial colors and flavors, and natural foods that contain aspirin-like compounds called salicylates. Within a few days, Tommy improved dramatically. He could sit down to eat and watch television, his temper tantrums greatly improved, and he obviously felt better about himself and his world because he was full of hugs and kisses.

Tommy started regular kindergarten and did well academically. But he still experienced times when he was overactive and anxious. We began to notice that certain natural foods that didn't contain salicylates bothered him as well. Eating homemade chocolate pudding made him extremely depressed and hysterical. After he ate homemade bread with added soy flour, Tommy was so hyperactive that he couldn't sit down for hours. These obvious, serious reactions triggered by eating common foods amazed us. Tommy also reacted to many chemicals in his environment.

When Tommy was twelve, he began to experience severe, chronic, migraine-like headaches. After we exhausted the traditional medical treatments, we consulted a nutritionally oriented physician experienced in diagnosing the biochemical causes of physical and behavioral problems. Special tests showed that Tommy had abnormal levels of the essential fatty acids in his blood. Supplementing Tommy's diet with special dietary oils not only cured his headaches, but also greatly improved his ability to deal calmly with the stresses of everyday life.

Tom was a delight as a teenager—calm, reasonable, happy, and hardworking. He graduated near the top of his class from a competitive high school and with high honors from a prestigious university. Now twenty-five years old, Tom attends graduate school. He has no trace of learning problems or ADHD!

Our second son, Jimmy, was born almost three years after Tommy. Like Tommy, Jimmy also suffered from severe colic. As a toddler, Jimmy often appeared tired and had dark circles under his eyes. He showed no signs of starting to talk. We took him to the university for hearing and language tests. His hearing was normal, but his language and gross-motor skills were at least a year and a half delayed. We were devastated. We enrolled him in a preschool program for children with language problems. Jimmy also experienced night terrors, which eventually began to occur during the day, too. The doctor prescribed Ritalin, but Jimmy didn't respond. Then we realized that certain foods "turned him on," too.

By the time Jimmy entered regular kindergarten, his speech had improved, although his development was still delayed. But he worked hard and learned to read and write without problems. His speech progressed rapidly. Special blood tests showed that Jimmy had low levels of many of the important fatty acids, and taking supplements greatly improved his health, behavior, and learning. Like Tom, Jim was a delight during his teenage years—calm, bright, insightful, and hardworking. He, too, was an honor student and finished near the top of his high school class. He excelled in college and was selected for Phi Beta Kappa. At twenty-two, Jim is healthy and happy.

There are many stories like Linda's. Also, personally, I have found that dietary changes dramatically improved my own emotional and physical health, and I have written three books to assist parents in changing their family's diet to help their children. Along this journey, I met William G. Crook, M.D., of Jackson, Tennessee. Dr. Crook has been working tirelessly since the mid-1950s to help hyperactive children, as well as children with other personality, behavior, and learning problems. He found that many of his patients felt and acted better when they identified and stopped eating common foods and additives. Dr. Crook and I had so many common interests that we teamed up to write a book to help more families.

My interest in the relationship of nutrition to behavior became so great that I returned to graduate school and recently earned my master of science degree in foods and nutrition from Purdue University. I loved my biochemistry classes, where I learned all about the metabolic pathways that require various nutrients—vitamins, minerals, amino acids, sugars, and essential fatty acids. For a food-science-class project, I studied the properties of natural food colorings compared with those of artificial colors. Studies have shown that many children with ADHD are "turned on" by artificial colors. I listened intently in one graduate seminar that dealt with recent studies reporting a direct relationship between food and additive sensitivities and hyperactivity.

For a research project, my professor and I studied nutritional factors, especially the essential fatty acids, in children with ADHD and children with normal behavior. Our results were published in the scientific literature, and our work with children with ADHD continues today. Through my research and my work, I have met many exhausted, frustrated parents who complained about the side effects of stimulant medication and asked, "Is there a better way to help my child?"

I have also created a website on the Internet, "The ADD/ADHD Online Newsletter." The purpose of this site is to disseminate information about diet and behavior, and how parents can help their children, often with little or no medication. More than 150,000 people have visited this website, and I have exchanged e-mails with thousands of desperate, concerned parents. Managing, controlling, and helping a hyperactive, inattentive child is a challenging and frustrating responsibility. In fact, it takes the patience of a saint!

I hope *12 Effective Ways to Help Your ADD/ADHD Child* will help you find better ways than medication to improve your child's behavior. To make things easier for you, I'm going to give you the nitty-gritty of how to identify the "pieces" in *your* child's "jigsaw puzzle." You don't have to tackle them all at once, just one at a time.

I wish I could promise every one of you that you'll find the missing pieces of your child's behavior puzzle with this book as your guide. I don't know if I can make that guarantee, but I can tell you that nutritionally oriented physicians who use these methods to help their patients have found that at least 75 percent of these children improved so much that they did not need medication. As new treatments and biological factors are identified, I'll keep you posted on my home page at http://www.nlci.com/nutrition.

A WORD ABOUT GENDER

Your child is certainly as likely to be a boy as a girl. However, the English language does not provide a genderless pronoun. To avoid the use of the awkward "he/she," the masculine pronouns "he," "him," and "his" are used when referring to a child, and the female pronouns "she," "her," and "hers" are used when referring to a parent, doctor, or teacher. This has been done in the interest of simplicity and clarity, and because many more boys than girls have ADD and ADHD.

INTRODUCTION

Johnny's mother, Louise, tried desperately to remain calm while she helped five-year-old Johnny get ready for school. But Johnny, who had recently been diagnosed as having ADHD, was running all over the house. He couldn't stand still to get his teeth brushed or his hair combed. He stood up to eat breakfast. When his mother put on his shoes, he took them off and threw them across the room. Ultimately, she would get him off to school, but much too often she received phone calls from his teacher at the end of the day.

His teacher complained that most days Johnny was all over the classroom. He chattered incessantly. He wandered around the classroom while the other children sat quietly listening to a story. He could not pay attention and was not learning his lessons. He cried and carried on when things didn't go his way. Finally the teacher reported, "I just can't deal with Johnny anymore. He requires more of my time than all of the children put together. It's not fair to the other children. Please talk to your doctor about medicating your child with Ritalin." Louise was crushed. She hated the idea of medicating her son to get him to behave, but what was she to do? Were there alternatives to drugs that might help her son?

The answer for her and so many other parents is a resounding "yes!" And in seeking an alternative, identifying and addressing biological factors that lead to symptoms of ADD or ADHD can be very helpful. That's the purpose of this book—to help you identify pieces of your child's behavior jigsaw puzzle.

In Part 1 of this book, "Understanding the Basics of ADD and ADHD," we'll look at what ADD and ADHD are, how they are diagnosed, and what the underlying causes may be. If you're planning to have more children, I'll give you some precautions to help avoid ADD/ADHD in a new baby.

In Part 2, "Twelve Ways to Help Your Child," I'll assist you in investigating which factors may be triggering your child's behavior and health problems. I'll present you with twelve ways you can help your child without drugs. Each chapter begins with a questionnaire to help you determine whether or not the following approach is likely to help your child. The first way is to improve the nutritional quality of your child's diet. If you put the wrong gas in your car, you could expect that the car might jerk, rattle, knock, and ultimately stop running. When you feed your child, you want to put the right fuel in his "tank."

The second way to help your child is to choose the sweeteners in his diet carefully. Many children with ADHD are bothered by sugar. But they also may have problems with artificial sweeteners, such as aspartame. We'll look at all the sweetening options, so you can make informed choices.

The third way to help your child is to track down hidden food allergies. Studies have shown that as many as 75 percent of children with ADHD are sensitive to one or more food colorings or common foods. Eliminating the foods that bother your child often dramatically improves his behavior and health.

A fourth way you can help your child is to add essential fatty acids to his diet. Essential fatty acids must be consumed in the diet because your body cannot make them. They play an especially important role in the central nervous system. The fifth way is to supplement his diet with the right vitamins and minerals in the right amounts.

The sixth helpful tactic is to look for a yeast connection. If your child has had many ear infections and antibiotics, he may have an overgrowth of the yeast *Candida albicans* in his intestines. You will need to supplement him with "good" bacteria to help displace the yeast, along with yeast-killing drugs and a low-sugar diet.

Way 7 for helping your child is to identify inhalant allergies. Some possible allergens include dust, mold, pollens, and animal dander. You may already know that your child is sensitive to one or more of these particles. What you may not know is that they can trigger behavior problems.

The eighth way to help your child is to identify chemicals in his environment that may be "turning him on." Common culprits include tobacco smoke, petroleum products, chlorine, and formaldehyde. The ninth way is to investigate lead and aluminum poisoning. Although this isn't the cause of symptoms in most children with ADHD, it is vital to the few who do have the problem.

The tenth and eleventh ways may seem a bit unconventional, but they have proven time and again to be effective. Way 10 involves the use of specially tinted lenses to correct perceptual problems. Children with reading difficulties may have problems with perception. Way 11 involves teaching children who skipped the crawling stage or did not crawl long enough to crawl again to mature an immature reflex. I'll tell you how to decide whether or not your child may benefit from special crawling exercises.

The twelfth way to help your child is to use biofeedback. I'll tell you what biofeedback is, how treatment works, and the pros and cons of biofeedback training.

In Part 3, "Helping Your Child Adjust to His New Diet," I will suggest ways to cope with any dietary changes you'll need to make. I'll give you grocery-shopping tips, show you how to make sense of food labels, and recommend what to substitute for the foods that trigger symptoms in your child. I'll also help you plan happy holidays. Finally, I'll give you sixty recipes that my family has enjoyed. They stress good nutrition and provide alternatives to sugary, fatty "treats."

In the appendices, I'll give you information about very important scientific studies to share with your doctor. I'll also present a sample elimination diet that one family used to identify the foods that triggered their son's problems. Finally, I'll give you a list of books and Internet sites where you can find more information.

With *12 Effective Ways to Help Your ADD/ADHD Child* as your guide, you will play detective. Remember, no one knows your child better than you do. Chances are, you won't solve your child's problems overnight, but you should know within a few weeks whether or not you're discovering important pieces to your child's behavior puzzle.

PART

1

Understanding the Basics of ADD and ADHD

WHAT ARE ADD
AND ADHD?

Your doctor or psychologist may have already labeled your child with the diagnosis of attention-deficit disorder (ADD) or attention-deficit hyperactivity disorder (ADHD). Your child's teacher may have complained that your child doesn't pay attention and isn't learning his lessons. She may have recommended that you see your doctor to inquire about the use of stimulant medication to help him focus his attention. Or, perhaps you suspect your child may have ADD or ADHD because he is having significant problems at home or in school.

ADD and ADHD are the most common behavioral disorders in children. Roughly 3 to 5 percent of the school-aged population in the United States is thought to have ADHD, although some experts think the percentage is much higher. A recent study reported that 18 to 20 percent of fifth-grade boys in two Virginia cities were taking stimulant drugs for ADHD. Boys are affected more commonly than girls, at a ratio estimated to be six to one or eight to one. About 20 to 30 percent of the children with ADHD have parents or siblings with ADHD. (The prevalence of ADD is thought to be lower.)

In this chapter, we will discuss what ADD and ADHD are. We will outline the symptoms of the two disorders, plus review some of the affiliated problems that children with ADD or ADHD may have. We will also describe what your initial visit to the doctor will most likely be like, and detail the traditional treatments that may be recommended.

Nutrition-oriented physicians have found that the techniques outlined in this book are effective for both ADHD and ADD, though ADD is a different psychological disorder from ADHD. However, most statistics and studies cited in this book refer to children with ADHD, unless stated otherwise.

SYMPTOMS OF ADD AND ADHD

There are a variety of symptoms generally associated with ADD and ADHD. While these symptoms are great in number, they can be organized into three general categories. First, children with ADD or ADHD are *inattentive*. When you give your child directions, you might as well be talking to the wall. Teachers complain that your child doesn't listen, is easily distracted, is "in another world," and doesn't finish his work. Second, children with ADHD are *impulsive*. They may blurt out answers in class without thinking and engage in dangerous activities without considering the consequences. Third, children with ADHD are *hyperactive*. In class, they may fidget and squirm. At home, they may constantly be restless and on the go. They may talk incessantly and show inappropriate levels of motor activity. As a consequence of these symptoms, children with ADD or ADHD often have severe problems at home, in school, and with peers.

Does your child have ADD or ADHD? As a first step, read the following statements and indicate whether they apply to your child "not at all," "just a little," "pretty much," or "very much." The statements are adapted from the criteria for diagnosing ADHD set by the American Psychiatric Association.[1] The problems should have persisted for at least six months, with the onset before the age of seven.

Inattention Problems

1. My child is easily distracted.
2. My child doesn't listen.
3. My child makes careless mistakes.
4. My child fails to finish his schoolwork and chores.
5. My child has trouble paying attention at school and in play situations.
6. My child loses things in school and at home.
7. My child avoids tasks that require attention.
8. My child has trouble organizing tasks and activities.
9. My child often is forgetful.

Hyperactivity/Impulsivity Problems

1. My child interrupts or intrudes.
2. My child talks incessantly.
3. My child engages in dangerous activities.
4. My child fidgets and squirms.
5. My child blurts out answers.
6. My child has problems playing quietly.
7. My child cannot remain seated.
8. My child is inattentive in school and at play.
9. My child is often "on the go" and acts as if "driven by a motor."
10. My child runs about or climbs excessively.

Of the inattention problems, how many of the nine statements did you rate as "pretty much" or "very much"? If six or more, your child may have an inattention problem. Of the hyperactivity/impulsivity problems, how many of the ten statements did you rate as "pretty much" or "very much"? If six or more, your child may have a hyperactivity problem. Some children have only inattention problems and are not hyperactive. They may have ADD. Other children have both inattention and hyperactivity problems. These children may have ADHD. What is important to remember is that all children have the symptoms of these problems at various times. What child doesn't not listen to instructions from time to time? What child doesn't engage in dangerous activities occasionally? What child doesn't fidget and squirm when bored? However, children with ADD or ADHD stand out because of the *frequency* and *severity* of their symptoms.

OTHER PROBLEMS OF ADD/ADHD CHILDREN

Unfortunately for their exhausted parents and frustrated teachers, children with ADHD are more likely to have other behavior disorders. For example, anywhere from 20 to 56 percent of children who have ADHD also have conduct disorder (CD).[2] A child with conduct disorder may tell lies, "con" others, initiate fights, show physical cruelty to people and animals, destroy other people's property, and bully others. More than half the children with ADHD also have symptoms of oppositional-defiant disorder (ODD). A child with ODD may argue frequently with adults, act vindictively, blame others for his mistakes, defy rules, and show anger and resentment. Anxiety disorder (AD) affects about 25 percent of children with ADD or ADHD. Children with anxiety disorder are significantly more anxious and worried than children with normal behavior. Other psychological problems include depression, Tourette syndrome, and obsessive-compulsive disorder (OCD).

In school, children with ADD or ADHD often perform poorly, have more specific learning disabilities, demonstrate deficient academic-achievement skills, experience more language and speech problems, and show delayed motor coordination. These children may be disruptive in the classroom and may even be suspended or expelled for their actions. About a third of the children repeat a grade. Approximately 30 to 40 percent require some type of special education. Anywhere from 10 to 35 percent fail to graduate from high school.[3]

At home, as you may know from firsthand experience, parents frequently have severe problems dealing with their ADD/ADHD children. The children's hyperactivity and excessive talking try everyone's patience, and getting them to do their homework in the evening is a Herculean task. These children may resist all efforts to settle down at night to go to sleep, even if they do not take stimulant medication. Their siblings may tire of coping with the trying behavior, and may resent the attention and special favors the ADD/ADHD children receive. Eating out and other family activities outside the home often end in disaster, with everyone angry at everyone else. If an ADD/ADHD child also has conduct disorder or oppositional-defiant disorder, the problems for the family members are multiplied. Not surprisingly, children with ADHD are more likely to have divorced parents. Then, the goal for the mothers and fathers becomes one of setting a structure and maintaining consistent discipline between the two households. Parenting a child with ADD or ADHD is a challenge for which no parent can be properly prepared. However, counseling and parenting classes can help harassed parents cope more effectively with their children's behavior.

Children with ADHD also have increased health problems, including more upper respiratory infections, allergies, asthma, ear infections, headaches, and stomachaches. They suffer more from bed-wetting.[4] These health problems are not new. As infants, 25 to 50 percent of children with ADHD were described as having "poor health during infancy." Children with ADHD are also more likely to have accidents and injuries.

The symptoms of ADD and ADHD also often persist into adulthood. It used to be thought that children outgrew their hyperactivity and other behavior problems. Now it's recognized that the problems of 50 to 80 percent of children with ADHD continue into adolescence and adulthood.[5] Earlier and current learning and behavior problems can have long-term adverse effects on academic and vocational achievement, social interaction, and emotional health. Adults may show low self-esteem, a low frustration level, poor listening skills, poor self-discipline, forgetfulness, marital problems, more traffic accidents—the list goes on.

SEE YOUR DOCTOR

A child with ADD or ADHD often has multiple problems, so he will need all the help he can get. Therefore, if you believe your child may have ADD or ADHD, take him to the doctor. A number of different professionals are qualified to make the diagnosis of ADD or ADHD. You may choose a clinical child psychologist or psychiatrist to be your team leader.

Your pediatrician can also make the diagnosis after gathering information from you and other professionals. Unfortunately, some doctors, because of time restrictions, listen for only ten or fifteen minutes to a parent and then prescribe medication. This is not the way to get the best help for a child.

If you suspect that your child has ADD or ADHD, the first step is to take him to his physician for a complete physical exam. Enlist the doctor's help in identifying the pieces of your child's puzzle. If the doctor is skeptical about some of the material in this book, you may find her more receptive if you show her the medical references discussed in Appendix A, "Scientific Studies for You and Your Doctor."

When you take your child to the doctor, the doctor will take a complete health history and perform a physical examination. Following are some of the areas your doctor (especially if she is interested in nutrition and the effect of foods on behavior and health) may explore with you and your child.

Health History

A good history gives a doctor more information than a physical examination, laboratory studies, allergy tests, and X rays. Of interest to the doctor are the mother's pregnancy history, the child's birth history, and his developmental milestones, allergies, illnesses, antibiotic usage, injuries, and everyday diet. Your doctor will also want to know about any medications, special diets, tutoring, behavior modification, or other treatment measures that you may have tried to help your child.

The doctor will also take a family medical history. She will ask if your child has any blood relatives (parents, siblings, grandparents, aunts, or uncles, living or deceased) who have suffered from allergies, including hay fever, asthma, eczema, hives, or a chronically stuffy, runny nose. She will ask if these relatives ever suffered from any food sensitivities and if they have ever been bothered by nervous or mental disorders, hyperactivity, inattention, impulsivity, conduct disorder, oppositional-defiant disorder, depression, or learning disorders. Have they suffered from arthritis, headaches, digestive problems, or autoimmune diseases?

As part of the pregnancy and birth history, the doctor will ask if the biological mother suffered any complications during her pregnancy. Did she undergo any physical or emotional distress? Did she consume alcohol, smoke cigarettes, or take drugs? What kind of diet did the mother consume during pregnancy? Were there any signs of fetal distress close to the time of delivery? Was the birth a normal vaginal delivery or a caesarian section? Were there any complications? Was the baby's color normal after birth? Did he have trouble breathing?

Your doctor will also question you about your child's health and behavior problems during infancy. She will ask what your child was like as an infant. If your child was breast-fed, she will ask if he had any problems with weight gain, colic, or spitting up. If he did, he may have been sensitive to foods his mother ate that entered her bloodstream and then her milk. If your child was bottle-fed, your doctor will ask if he had any difficulties with his formula, weight gain, colic, spitting up, or vomiting. If he did, he may have been sensitive to cow's milk or soymilk, depending on the formula he was fed. The doctor will also ask if he had such digestive problems as bloating, diarrhea, or stomachaches. Did he have frequent respiratory problems such as colds, noisy breathing, repeated ear infections, or a stuffy, runny nose? Did he take repeated courses of antibiotics for ear infections? Was he a difficult baby? Was he irritable, overactive, or a poor sleeper?

The doctor will also ask about your child's current behavior and health problems. She will want to know if he has hay fever, asthma, hives, eczema, or a chronically stuffy, itchy, runny nose. Does he have digestive problems such as diarrhea, constipation, or stomachaches? Does he have frequent headaches? Does he complain of muscle aches? Is he often tired even though he had a good night's sleep? Does he have dark circles or puffiness around his eyes? Is his complexion pale and washed-out? Is his behavior worse in some seasons of the year than others? If he is more than three years old, does he still wet the bed frequently? No matter what age he is, does he have a Dr. Jekyll–Mr. Hyde personality—happy and well-behaved one minute, irritable and bouncing off the walls the next?

Your doctor will also ask what your child is like in school. She will want to know about his school performance. She will want to know if he has good days and bad days in school. If he has good and bad days, what might be different in his diet on the bad days? The doctor will also want to gather information from your child's teacher, including the results of any standardized achievement tests, a Teacher Behavior Rating question-naire, evidence of academic achievement, and comments about the child's behavior in class, at recess, and with peers.

Your doctor will also want to review your child's psychologist's report. If you and/or your child were interviewed by a psychologist, and if the psychologist administered any behavior and learning tests, your doctor will be interested in the results. For example, your child may have been given computer tests that measure attention and impulsivity.

Your child's dietary concerns will also be of interest to the doctor. Is your child a picky eater? Does his behavior worsen when he doesn't eat on time? Are there any foods you know that "turn him on" or make him sick? Does he crave certain foods, especially sugary ones? Is he a "sugarholic"? Does his behavior or health worsen around holiday times when he con-sumes more sugary foods and artificial colors and flavors? Does he have excessive thirst or frequent urination?

All of these questions will help your doctor put together a profile of your child that can help her determine important pieces of your child's puzzle.

Physical Examination

The second part of your child's examination will be a physical checkup. First, the doctor will appraise the child's overall appearance. Does he look happy or unhappy, calm or jittery, clumsy or well coordinated? How well does he write his name and read from an age-appropriate book? Does he have speech problems?

Your doctor may look for the characteristic signs of allergy. Some of these are:

- A pale color (in the absence of iron-deficiency anemia)
- Red earlobes or cheeks
- Allergic "shiners" (dark shadows or wrinkles under the eyes)
- A congested nose, with or without a crease across it
- Allergic gape (the tendency to keep the mouth open because the nose is stopped up)
- Chapped lips or patches of rash on the face or other parts of the body

- "Geographic tongue" or "wandering rash" (spots that make the tongue look like a map and that tend to move around)[6]

Next, the doctor will check your child from head to toe. Are his skin and hair dull and dry? Does he have dandruff? Are his fingernails brittle or broken? Does he have small, hard bumps on the backs of his arms or on his thighs? Except in the occasional troubled child who suffers from asthma, eczema, or fluid in his ears, the remainder of the physical examination will most likely be normal.

Careful vision and hearing tests are also important. Ask your doctor to check your child's hearing, and consult an ophthalmologist or optometrist to have his vision assessed. Children with hearing loss or poor vision have trouble paying attention and learning. One three-year-old girl was a terror until her new doctor screened her for hearing problems and found a significant hearing loss, which was easily treated. The little girl is now a bright, happy toddler.

In children with behavior problems, laboratory tests for iron deficiency and thyroid dysfunction may be indicated. Although most children with ADD or ADHD do not have these problems, identifying these abnormalities can be crucial for the few who do. Again, different children have different puzzle pieces.

Marginal Iron Deficiency   Iron deficiency is the most common nutritional deficiency in both the United States and the world. In children, the most common cause is low dietary iron intake. Iron deficiency can lead to behavior problems, decreased intellectual performance, and lowered resistance to infection.[7] Iron-deficient children are also at a higher risk for lead poisoning.

To determine if your child has a marginal iron deficiency, begin by answering the following questions:

1. Is your child pale?
2. Is your child tired?
3. Is your child inattentive?
4. Is your child irritable?

5. Is your child performing poorly in school?
6. Is your child a large milk consumer? (Milk contains little iron, and the calcium in it inhibits the absorption of iron from other foods.)
7. Is your child a poor consumer of red meats?
8. Is your child a picky eater?

If you answered yes to any of the foregoing questions, ask your doctor to test for a marginal iron deficiency. The best test to assess iron status measures the serum-ferritin level, an indicator of the iron stores in the body. If the serum-ferritin level is low, the iron store in the liver is depleted, indicating that the total-body storage of iron is also low. Even if your child does not have iron-deficiency anemia, low iron stores can affect his behavior and school performance.

If the test shows that your child is deficient in iron, your doctor may prescribe an iron supplement, and she certainly will encourage you to give your child more iron-rich foods. Here are some foods high in iron that children enjoy:

Beef liver, 3 ounces, 5.3 milligrams of iron
Beef pot roast, 3 ounces, 2.0 milligrams of iron
Turkey, dark meat, 3 ounces, 2.0 milligrams of iron
Tuna, 3 ounces, 1.9 milligrams of iron
Green peas, ½ cup, 1.8 milligrams of iron
Hamburger, lean, 3 ounces, 1.8 milligrams of iron
Chicken drumstick, 1 average, 1.0 milligram of iron
Egg, 1 large, .07 milligram of iron
Banana, 1 medium, 0.9 milligram of iron
Potato, baked, 1 medium, 0.7 milligram of iron
Peanut butter, 2 tablespoons, 0.6 milligram of iron
Whole wheat bread, 1 slice, 0.5 milligram of iron

Consuming supplements and iron-rich foods with foods that contain vitamin C enhances iron absorption. The Recommended Dietary Allowance (RDA) for children aged one to ten is 10 milligrams of iron. For older children, the iron RDA is 12 milligrams for boys and 15 milligrams for girls.

Do not give your child iron supplements unless blood tests show he is iron-deficient. Too much iron in the system can interfere with the absorption of other important minerals. Keep all iron supplements out of the reach of young children to prevent iron poisoning, which can be life-threatening.

Thyroid Problems   Thyroid hormone is necessary for normal brain development. New research reports that a few children with ADHD who show symptoms of thyroid disease or have a family history of thyroid disease (especially generalized resistance to thyroid hormone) should be screened for thyroid abnormalities using a blood test for free thyroxine index and thyrotropin.[8]

In a recent study, doctors gave thyroid hormone to eight children with ADHD and generalized resistance to thyroid hormone (GRTH), and to nine children with ADHD and no thyroid problems.[9] Among the children with no thyroid problems, seven did not change, one improved, and one became worse. Among the children with ADHD and GRTH, five of the eight children improved.

Dr. Mary Ann Block, in her book *No More Ritalin*, commented:

Too much focus on the psychological side distracts us from looking for the real problem, which is often more physiological than psychological. Too often I have seen children who have had an expensive psychological evaluation without a proper medical workup. Since I think that such conditions as low blood sugar, allergies, and even thyroid dysfunction can contribute to ADHD symptoms and behavioral changes, the child should be medically evaluated and treated before jumping to the conclusion that the problem is only psychological. But this appears to be done rarely. Last year I diagnosed four children with hyperthyroidism in four months. All of the children had been diagnosed with ADHD. When the thyroid problem was addressed, the symptoms (which had been called ADHD) resolved.[10]

Thyroid dysfunction is probably not the reason for your child's behavior, but it may be. Remember that what you and your doctor do not look for may not be found!

TRADITIONAL TREATMENT

Doctors are trained to diagnose and label diseases. Once they've labeled the disease, they can prescribe drugs, surgery, or counseling. If your doctor labels your child as having ADD or ADHD, she may recommend or prescribe drugs to relieve the symptoms.

Stimulant drugs are the most commonly prescribed medications for ADD and ADHD. The most popular ones are Ritalin (methylphenidate), Cylert (pemoline), Adderall, and Dexedrine (dextroamphetamine). Another group of drugs used to treat children with ADHD who don't respond to stimulant medications or who have other psychiatric problems are antidepressants such as amitriptyline and imipramine. A third type of drug is also being prescribed to help ADD/ADHD children. This group includes the antihypertensive (blood-pressure-lowering) drugs such as Clonidine (catapres), which improve behavior in some children with ADHD.[11] Clonidine is a potent drug. What parents usually don't realize is that Clonidine alone or in combination with Ritalin has been associated with three deaths in children.[12] At present, there's controversy over whether children taking both Clonidine and a stimulant drug need a baseline electrocardiogram (EKG) and subsequent EKGs to monitor the effects of the drugs. The children's pulse and blood pressure may also need to be monitored. However, other researchers and physicians are not convinced of a link between Clonidine and the three deaths, and do not perform EKGs.[13] One thing is clear: Clonidine and any other drugs that ADD/ADHD children take should *never* be stopped abruptly without the help of a doctor. As you can see, these drugs are powerful and should not be used without careful consideration of the benefits versus the possible complications.

What are the pros and cons of giving your child stimulant medication? First, the pros:

- They are easy to use and work quickly, so you'll know soon if they're going to help or not. They improve both behavior and school performance. They are relatively inexpensive.

- They have been used for many years, so doctors have a lot of experience in prescribing them.
- Medication may provide relief for a child who is about to be expelled from school or whose family structure is falling apart.

What are the cons of giving stimulant medication and the reasons to look for other solutions?

- About 20 to 30 percent of children with ADHD do not respond to stimulant medication.
- According to the *Physicians' Desk Reference*, a doctors' guide to prescription drugs, "Ritalin should never be used in children under six years since safety and efficacy in this age group have not been established."[14] The same applies to Cylert.
- In a few children, Cylert causes liver problems, so a baseline liver-function test is required, with subsequent follow-up tests after the medicine has been started.
- Stimulant drugs may decrease children's appetites, reducing the intake of foods containing essential nutrients.
- Some children may be especially difficult to manage late in the day and in the evening, when the medication has worn off ("behavior rebound"). This can be a trial for families who are already exhausted and stressed at the end of the day. Children on stimulant drugs may have trouble falling asleep.
- A few children on stimulant medication complain of frequent stomachaches and headaches.
- About 1 to 2 percent of children on stimulant medication develop tics.
- Many parents dislike even the thought of medicating their children. One worried mom recently wrote: "I find myself *very* reluctant to 'drug' a six-year-old child. I'm looking for better ways to help my child."

- Many children do not like taking medication. They are embarrassed to go to the nurse's office at school to get their noon dose. They may mistakenly view the drug as a "dumb pill." Some children don't like how they feel on medication. Teenagers often refuse to take medication.

- Surprisingly, long-term studies of children who take stimulant drugs do not show that these children are better off than those who do not take medication. They do not show long-term improvement in academic achievement, a decrease in antisocial behavior, or a decrease in arrest rates. Reading skills, athletic skills, social skills, and performance on learning tests do not improve long-term.[15]

Furthermore, medication does not answer the important questions: *Why* is my child hyperactive? *Why* can't he pay attention? *Why* is he so impulsive? *What* is causing these behaviors? Some people like to compare Ritalin to insulin. These substances are really quite different, however. Insulin is a naturally occurring hormone, and in some ways, diabetics are "insulin deficient." No one has a Ritalin deficiency. Ritalin is not a naturally occurring substance. Taking Ritalin for ADD or ADHD is like taking aspirin for frequent, severe headaches: the aspirin helps the headache, but it does not address the basic, underlying cause of the pain. Ritalin does not "fix" an ADD/ADHD child's problems.

The dramatically increasing use of Ritalin concerns many doctors, psychologists, educators, and parents. Since 1990, the use of Ritalin has risen two and a half times. More than 1.3 million children take Ritalin regularly. Yet, medication should *never* be used alone. A multidisciplinary approach is essential. The parents of ADD/ADHD children should be given training in behavior-modification techniques to enable them to more effectively rear these hard-to-raise children. Teachers, school counselors, and school principals should be actively involved in finding ways to improve these children's learning and behavior.

If your doctor recommends that your child take Ritalin or another drug, discuss your concerns with her. If you decide to go the medication route for now, remember that you are not ruling out looking for the underlying factors that this book addresses. If your child is currently taking stimulant drugs, don't halt them without consulting your physician. Search for the pieces that will complete your child's puzzle of a happy, healthy, well-adjusted child.

CAUSES OF ADD AND ADHD

Although exactly what goes awry in the brains of children with ADD and ADHD is not known, there appear to be multiple biological factors in the development of the disorder. Researchers are using exciting new methods to learn more about the brain, including the noninvasive and painless magnetic resonance imaging (MRI) scans to study the structure of the brain and positron emission tomography (PET) to study brain metabolism, as well as molecular biology to identify genes associated with ADHD. Here are some of the potential causes of ADD/ADHD that have been identified to date.

BRAIN PHYSIOLOGY

Through the use of new technology, scientists have noted some minor differences between the brains of children with ADHD and the brains of other children. MRI helps researchers view the brain. In some studies, researchers have determined that the right side of the brain is generally smaller in children with ADHD than in those who do not have ADHD. This may be important because certain neurotransmitters that affect mental and emotional functioning are located in this portion of the brain.

Using PET, scientists are able to observe the brain's function. With this imaging technique, researchers have been able to measure the level of the brain's activity while study subjects were trying to memorize a list of words. They did this by measuring glucose levels with PET scans. Glucose is the brain's main source of energy, so they could determine the brain's activity level by measuring how much glucose was used. The researchers discovered that in the brains of those with ADHD, the area that controls attention used less glucose than in the brains of those who did not have ADHD. Scientists are now trying to determine why this is so.

BRAIN TRAUMA

Doctors have known for years that children with brain damage due to injury or serious brain infection may show inattention and hyperactivity. Mothers of children with ADHD had a greater incidence of complications during pregnancy, during labor, or at birth. Furthermore, children of mothers who smoked, drank alcohol, or took illegal drugs during pregnancy have a greater incidence of ADHD. For these reasons, minor head injury, unhealthy pregnancies, childbirth complications, and undetectable brain damage have been investigated as possible causes of ADD/ADHD. However, while a significant percentage of children with the above histories have problems with attention and hyperactivity, most children with ADHD do not have brain injury, a history of brain infection, or mothers who engaged in these activities. So these do not appear to be very common causes of ADD/ADHD.

GENETICS

There also appears to be a strong genetic component to ADHD. If a mother or father has ADHD, a child has a 57 percent chance of also having the disorder.[1] If a sibling has ADHD, a child has a 32 percent risk of having ADHD. Among twins with ADHD, identical twins are more likely to have ADHD than fraternal twins. However, not every identical twin with ADHD has a twin with ADHD, so genes aren't everything.

So far, three genes are suspected of playing a role in ADHD in some children. One gene is the thyroid receptor gene on chromosome 3. But this appears to be a rare cause of ADHD, affecting only a handful of children; but it is a critical factor for children who do have this genetic problem. The second gene contains the codes for a transporter for the important neurotransmitter dopamine. Interestingly, this is the site where Ritalin is thought to act in the brain. The third gene contains the gene for a dopamine receptor. Undoubtedly, more genes will be discovered that play roles in ADD and ADHD.

A number of genetic disorders often cause symptoms of ADHD. For example, fragile X syndrome is the most common genetic cause of mental retardation. Almost all boys with fragile X syndrome have severe hyperactivity and inattention. About 35 percent of girls with this disorder show symptoms of ADHD. Another genetic abnormality is sex-chromosomal abnormalities. For example, females with Turner's syndrome often have ADHD. Males with XYY syndrome often have learning problems and exhibit aggression. Tourette syndrome is a genetic disorder characterized by motor and vocal tics. ADHD is common in children with Tourette syndrome.

ENVIRONMENTAL FACTORS

Environmental factors also play a role in the cause of ADD/ADHD, and as you've probably picked up on by now, I strongly believe these are among the most important factors. Environmental toxins, like lead and aluminum, are known to disrupt some brain processes and brain development.

Exposure to such toxins could lead to symptoms of ADD/ADHD. See Way 9 to learn more about this. Likewise, food and inhalant allergies may play a role in the development of ADD/ADHD. See Way 3 and Way 7 for more on allergies and ADD/ADHD. The majority of this book focuses on environmental factors and their causal role in these disorders.

•

Diagnostic labels such as ADD and ADHD help doctors and patients communicate. They are also important at school, where this diagnosis opens the door to special-education programs. What's even more important is looking at the whole child. Two children may have the same symptom—hyperactivity—for entirely different reasons. One child may have sensitivities to artificial colors while another child may have lead poisoning. Likewise, two children may have identical biological abnormalities but show completely different symptoms. One child who is sensitive to milk may suffer from fatigue and irritability while another child who is also sensitive to milk wets the bed.

In Part 2, I will try to help you determine the cause of your child's ADD/ADHD and provide you with options for eliminating the causes.

AN OUNCE OF
PREVENTION

I must first make it clear that parents are not the cause of their child's ADD/ADHD. My intent in writing this chapter was not to place the blame on the parents of a child with ADD/ADHD. It does appear, however, that certain factors present during pregnancy can contribute to a child's development of ADD/ADHD. And, as the old saying goes, "An ounce of prevention is worth a pound of cure." Parents of a child with ADD/ADHD who are planning to have another child would do well to heed this advice. It's much easier to be cautious before and after birth than it is to control a child's behavior and health problems after they develop. As noted previously, ADD and ADHD run in families. Part of this may be because of the relationship between allergy and ADD/ADHD (see Way 3, Way 7) and the fact that allergic tendencies are inherited. Or perhaps special needs for certain nutrients are inherited. Also, there may be environmental factors at work—too much lead in the home, chemical exposures, or a poor diet. Of course, there are many children with ADHD who have no relatives with the disorder. You can't change your genes, but there are steps you can take that may improve your odds of having a child without attention problems.

NUTRITION

Excellent nutrition prior to and during pregnancy and lactation is essential. Ideally, both the mother and father will have been practicing good nutrition for years before conception. But it's never too late to start. What you eat during pregnancy will affect the emotional, mental, and physical development of your child. You need to keep yourself in optimal condition.

Eating a well-balanced, varied diet, avoiding lots of sugar, caffeine, salt, and additives, and taking vitamin and mineral supplements as prescribed by your doctor may help you feel better and benefit your unborn child. Pregnant women should take in daily at least three servings of milk, yogurt, and cheese (four servings if the pregnant woman is a teenager); three servings of lean meat, poultry, fish, dry beans, eggs, and nuts; three to five servings of vegetables; two to three servings of fruits; six to eleven servings of whole grain bread, cereal, rice, and pasta; and plenty of omega-3 fatty acids (the "good" fats).

Follow the guidelines for the Food Guide Pyramid outlined in Way 1. If you can't drink milk or don't like it, talk to your doctor about calcium supplements. If you are considering getting pregnant, be sure to get enough folic acid, one of the B vitamins, in your diet or as supplements. Sufficient amounts of folic acid help prevent devastating birth defects such as spina bifida.

Get plenty of nutritious fats—omega-3 fatty acids—in your diet before the pregnancy (to build up supplies in your fat tissue), during pregnancy, and during lactation. Omega-3 fatty acids are critical in the formation and development of the brain and retina of the eye. Foods rich in omega-3 fatty acids include flax and flaxseed oil, cold-pressed soy and canola oils, walnuts and cold-pressed walnut oil, tofu, beans (northern, soy, kidney, and navy), cod liver oil, and coldwater fish (fresh tuna, salmon, sardines, mackerel, and herring).

TOBACCO SMOKE

Avoid all contact with tobacco smoke. Mothers who smoke are more likely to have children with ADHD than mothers who don't. Mothers who smoke are more likely to have low-birth-weight babies. Don't let anyone smoke in your house or car.

ALCOHOL

Don't drink at all while you're pregnant or planning to become pregnant. Drinking alcohol can lead to a low-birth-weight baby and neurological damage. It's not known what level of alcohol is safe (if any) so it's advised to avoid all alcohol. That means no beer, wine, or hard alcohol. Children born with fetal alcohol syndrome have physical abnormalities, poor growth, and mental retardation. They may also be irritable and hyperactive and experience learning problems. In 1981, the Centers for Disease Control and Prevention recommended total abstinence from alcohol during pregnancy. Yet a recent survey found that between 1991 and 1995 the casual drinking of alcohol increased by 30 percent. Frequent drinking also increased. Your child's future is at stake—don't drink.

DRUGS, CAFFEINE, AND ASPARTAME

All drugs, both legal and illegal, prescription and over-the-counter, should be avoided unless prescribed by your doctor. Caffeine is considered a drug, so avoid all caffeinated beverages—coffee, tea, cocoa, and caffeine-containing soft drinks. Chocolate also contains caffeine. Avoid over-the-counter medications containing caffeine. To be on the safe side, avoid foods sweetened with aspartame during pregnancy and lactation.

STRESS

If possible, you should avoid stress. Stress before, during, or after birth may increase the likelihood of future allergies. Avoiding stress may be a challenge for you if you already have a child with ADHD!

BREAST-FEEDING

Breast really is best! The American Academy of Pediatrics recommends that mothers nurse their infants for at least six months, and preferably throughout the first year of life. Breast-feeding your child for any length of time benefits your baby.

Healthy People 2000, a federally funded program, has set a goal of 75 percent of women nursing their babies when they leave the hospital, and 50 percent still nursing their babies after six months. They have a long way to go. Currently only 50 percent of mothers in the United States nurse their babies in the hospital, while 20 percent are still nursing at six months.[1]

Why is "breast best"? Breast milk is specifically designed for human babies, just as cow's milk is specifically designed for calves. Human breast milk is very different from cow's milk, and as hard as they try, scientists cannot produce an infant formula identical to breast milk. Breast is best for your baby for a number of reasons:

- Breast milk is always fresh. It is already sterile. The temperature is just right. It's cheap and requires no preparation.
- Breast milk is easily digested. Breast-fed babies don't become constipated or thirsty because the breast milk provides all the water they need.
- Breast milk contains antibodies that pass from the mother to the baby to protect him against allergies and illnesses. Breast-fed babies have fewer gastrointestinal and respiratory infections and fewer ear infections.
- The first fluid to appear after birth is colostrum. It contains antibodies, white blood cells, and growth factors, which are ab-

sorbed into the baby's bloodstream because their intestines are porous and immature. These protect the infant from gastrointestinal disease. Bifidus factor in the breast milk encourages the growth of healthy, intestinal bacteria *Lactobacillus bifidus*. These bacteria limit the growth of toxic bacteria. The bifidus factor is not present in formulas.

- Several important proteins are present in breast milk. Lactalbumin, the primary protein in breast milk, eases digestion. Lactoferrin proteins bind iron, which is then easily absorbed. This reduces the growth of iron-dependent bacteria that may cause diarrhea. Taurine, an amino acid, aids indirectly in the digestion of fats and is important in brain development.

- Breast milk contains critical long-chain omega-6 and omega-3 fatty acids. (Way 4 will give you more information about essential fatty acids.) GLA, an omega-6 fatty acid, is a precursor for certain hormone-like chemicals that help delay the onset of allergies. Omega-3 fatty acids are crucial in building brain tissues, nerves, and the retina of the eye. At present, GLA and long chain fatty acids are not added to formulas.

- Breast milk has a high concentration of complex carbohydrates (oligosaccharides and glycoconjugates), which inhibit infection.

- Like iron, the zinc in breast milk is more easily absorbed than zinc in formulas. Zinc plays an important role in the developing immune system.

- Preterm infants who were fed breast milk had significantly higher IQs (8 points) than preterm infants fed formula.[2] The effect wasn't due to breast-feeding itself because the infants receiving breast-milk were fed the milk by bottle.

- Breast-fed babies have better cheekbone development and fewer speech problems because of sucking at the breast.

- Breast-feeding encourages the creation of a special bond between mother and child.

There are also benefits for you with breast-feeding. The baby's sucking at the breast after birth causes your uterus to contract and leads to less blood loss. The sucking also helps the uterus return to its pre-pregnancy shape and size. Breast-feeding burns up a lot of calories, so your weight returns to normal more quickly. Breast-feeding also seems to reduce the risk of developing breast cancer by 20 percent.

Women who work outside the home can still breast-feed by expressing their milk and refrigerating it until a caregiver can give the baby the bottle of breast milk. This takes a lot of dedication on the part of the mother. While the goal is to breast-feed until the baby is six months old, any breast-feeding that you can provide helps the baby. If you have problems breast-feeding or have questions, you can contact your local La Leche League or La Leche League on the Internet. La Leche League is an international organization that supports mothers who choose to breast-feed and provides lots of helpful information about breast-feeding.

While breast-feeding, continue to watch your diet closely—you are still eating for two. What you eat will affect your baby. If your baby develops colic or spits up frequently, you should keep a diet diary, recording whatever you eat and drink. See if there is any relationship between a change in your diet and your baby's reactions. A prime suspect is cow's milk, but eggs, chocolate, citrus fruits, and wheat also commonly present problems. If the mother is sensitive to a food she eats, the baby may also react. But the baby may also react to a food the mother is not sensitive to. Think twice before switching a colicky, sickly baby from breast milk. The very babies who are fussy and irritable on breast milk often do even worse on formula. Talk to your doctor about what is best for you and your baby.

SOLID FOODS

Don't be in a rush to start your baby on solid foods. Early introduction of solid foods may lead to allergies, as the proteins in them are foreign to the baby's immune system. Many doctors believe that infants (particularly ones with allergic parents or siblings) should be exclusively breast-fed for six months. Introduction of any solid foods should be postponed. This may make you feel uneasy, and you may be criticized by relatives and friends who all started solids earlier. Your baby doesn't need these foods in the early months. The longer you wait, the better the chances your child won't become sensitive to the new foods. Feeding solids in these early months does not help your baby to sleep through the night.

If you are tempted to speed up this schedule, listen to this advice from the Allergy Information Association of Canada:

The baby doesn't need it. It is you that needs the variety. Fast feeding is beneficial to the baby food companies, not to your baby. Fast feeding is a symptom of our hurry, flurry world. Above all, remember that how you feed the baby in the first year will affect him all his life. He will be what he eats.[3]

Should you buy baby food or make your own? Either way, there are pros and cons. You'll have to decide what's best for you, your lifestyle, and your baby. Fortunately, baby food companies have made an effort to improve their products by removing salt, preservatives, and artificial coloring and flavorings, as well as by reducing or eliminating sugar. But some products do contain sweeteners, so always read labels carefully. Juices may contain sugar or corn sweeteners.

According to the Academy of Pediatrics, children younger than a year should not drink cow's milk. Between ages one and two, children should be fed whole milk—they actually need the extra fat for normal development. After age two, children can drink 1- or 2-percent milk.

Once your child is old enough to eat what the rest of the family is eating, be sure to keep his diet nutritious and free from sugary, nutritionally empty snacks. In general, children who start life on the best foods, and continue eating them in their early years, won't crave sweets and junk foods. They'll grow up demanding good, nutritious foods.

•

There are no guarantees that these steps will keep your new child free of physical and behavioral problems. You can't change your genes, but you can change your child's internal and external environments. The stakes for your child are high and worth the extra effort.

PART

2

Twelve
Ways to
Help Your
Child

WAY 1.
IMPROVE YOUR
CHILD'S DIET

A nutritionally optimal diet may not seem important, but in reality, it is critical. The body resembles the most amazing chemical factory and warehouse ever designed. It manufactures, processes, and stores more than 100,000 different chemicals. To make these chemicals, it imports only about forty to fifty raw materials, chemicals it can't make by itself or in sufficient quantities—ten essential amino acids, two essential fatty acids, twenty to thirty minerals, twelve or so vitamins, water, glucose, and fiber. If the body doesn't take in enough of these raw materials and absorb them adequately, it can't function optimally. As a result, some of the assembly lines may perform erratically or shut down. Garbage in, garbage out!

If your child's breakfast is a doughnut or sugary cereal; his lunch potato chips, a bologna sandwich, and a Twinkie; his dinner fast food; and his snacks candy, chips, soft drinks, or fruit punches, his diet is not that unusual in today's hectic world. I know, because I computerized the three-day diet records of 100 children as part of a research study at Purdue University.

If your child consumes this "average" diet, you may find him experiencing a dramatic improvement in his behavior and health upon improvement in his food selections.

To help determine how your child's diet rates, answer yes or no to the following questions:

1. Does your child eat six to eleven servings of bread, cereal, rice, and pasta every day?
2. Does your child eat whole-grain breads and cereals, and brown rice?
3. Does your child eat unsweetened or only slightly sweetened cereals?
4. Does your child eat at least five servings of fruits and vegetables every day?
5. Does your child drink 100 percent pure unsweetened fruit juice (not fruit punch)?
6. Does your child eat two to three servings of lean meat, poultry, fish, eggs, dry beans, and nuts every day?
7. Does your child consume no soft drinks, candy, or foods high in added sugars?
8. Does your child consume nuts, seeds, and pure cold-pressed vegetable oil (especially soy or canola oil) every day?
9. Does your child consume only small amounts of saturated, hydrogenated, and partially hydrogenated fats?
10. Does your child consume two to three servings of low-fat milk and dairy products (or take calcium supplements) every day?

If you answered yes to most of the above questions, congratulations! It's not easy to feed a family a nutritionally optimal diet in today's hectic world. However, if you answered no to many of the questions, this chapter will show you some ways in which you can improve your child's diet while improving his health.

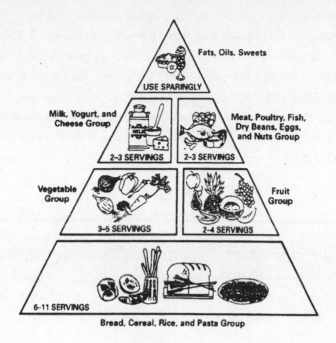

Food Guide Pyramid

FOOD GUIDE PYRAMID

To improve your child's diet and health, you don't have to make changes that are time-consuming or expensive. In fact, all you have to do is follow the Food Guide Pyramid that you've been seeing on television and on some food labels (see above). You've probably been intending to improve your family's diet for some time anyway—now is the ideal time.

Offer your child *variety*—different fruits, vegetables, grains, meats, fish, and so on. For example, a variety of fruits might include citrus fruits, apples, pears, pineapple, melons, peaches, nectarines, and kiwis. Variety will help ensure that your child gets all the nutrients he needs for good health. It also reduces his likelihood of developing an allergy to a food he eats repeatedly.

Use the Food Guide Pyramid as a map to what your child should eat each day. At the base of the pyramid are bread, cereal, rice, and pasta. The most servings of these foods are needed each day. At the tip of the pyramid are fats, oils, and sweets. These should be used sparingly and chosen carefully. In between are fruits; vegetables; lean meat, poultry, fish, eggs, dry beans, and nuts; and milk, yogurt, and cheese. Keep in mind that preschool children need the same variety of foods as older family members, but they can eat smaller servings of them. (Note, however, that preschoolers still require two cups of milk a day.)

Bread, Cereal, Rice, and Pasta

Your child should eat six to eleven servings of bread, cereal, rice, and pasta every day. Select whole-grain (wheat, rye, oat, rice, barley, millet, and corn) flours, breads, and crackers; unsweetened cereals; and brown rice. These foods supply the B vitamins, vitamin E, iron, magnesium, trace minerals, complex carbohydrates, incomplete protein, and fiber. A serving is one slice of bread, one ounce of ready-to-eat cereal, or one-half cup of cooked cereal, rice, or pasta.

Many cereals featured and promoted during children's television programs are 40 percent or more sugar and contain artificial colors and preservatives. A 14-ounce box of such a cereal may contain 50 or more teaspoons of sugar. (See the table on page 50 for the sugar content of many popular cereals.) In the experience of many nutritionally oriented physicians, sugar is a major cause of behavioral disorders in children, including hyperactivity, inappropriate drowsiness, and short attention span.[1] So while it is important that your child consume grain foods, including cereals, be sure to choose his cereal carefully, avoiding those loaded with sugar and artificial ingredients. But keep in mind that many children with ADD/ADHD do better with fewer carbohydrates and more protein foods.

Fruits and Vegetables

After bread, cereal, rice, and pasta, your child should consume fruits and vegetables in the greatest quantities. Aim for at least two to four servings of fruits and three to five servings of vegetables each day. This goal can be reached with orange juice for breakfast; vegetable soup for lunch; veggies, such as carrots and cherry tomatoes, and fruits for snacks; and a salad at dinner made with dark leafy greens, cabbage, and carrots, with salad dressing made with "good" fats. Apples, bananas, pears, grapes, orange sections, strawberries, and unsweetened applesauce all make easy, tasty, naturally sweet desserts and snacks. How much is a serving? One medium apple, banana, or orange; a half cup of cooked or canned fruit; and three-quarters of a cup of 100 percent pure unsweetened fruit juice all constitute one serving. Sorry, fruit pies don't count because of their high sugar and fat contents! One serving of vegetables is one cup of raw leafy vegetables; a half cup of cooked, chopped, or raw vegetables; or three-quarters of a cup of vegetable juice. No, potato chips and French fries don't count because of their high fat content.

Fruits provide important amounts of vitamins A and C, minerals, complex carbohydrates, and fiber. Give your child whole fruits. They are higher in fiber than fruit juices. Count only 100 percent fruit juice as fruit. Fruit punches and most fruit drinks contain only a little juice and lots of added sugar. Limit 100 percent fruit juices to one and a half cups a day so that your child has room for other nutritious foods. Some juices are more nutritious than others. Tomato, grapefruit, and orange juices are especially nutritious. Some children with ADD or ADHD have problems drinking pure fruit juice, especially on an empty stomach. Some tolerate whole fruits or juices better if they are consumed with a snack that includes a protein food. Some children need to avoid all fruit juices. A whole fruit may be tolerated better than fruit juice because the fiber helps slow the absorption of the fruit sugar. Apple juice has almost no fiber, applesauce has one and a half grams of fiber in a half cup, and a medium apple has three grams.

Vegetables provide vitamins, iron, calcium, trace minerals, complex carbohydrates, and fiber. Some fruits and vegetables, especially those that are orange or dark green, are more nutritious than others. You'll want to include these "stars" frequently in your child's diet. Among the best fruits and vegetables to include are blackberries, cantaloupe, grapefruit, kiwis, mangos, oranges, papayas, peaches, strawberries, tomatoes, broccoli, carrots, collard greens, kale, red peppers, spinach, and sweet potatoes.

If your child is like many of his peers, he may look at vegetables and say, "Yuck! No way! They're green." Many kids do not eat their vegetables (and neither do their parents!), and one-quarter of all the "vegetables" eaten by children are French fries. Here are some tips on how to get your child to eat more vegetables:

- Be a good role model. If you eat your veggies with pleasure, your child will be more inclined to eat them, too.
- Use hunger as a weapon. Provide a platter of raw veggies as an afternoon or evening snack for friends and family. Try a tasty vegetable dip to help sell the vegetables to finicky kids. (For a good recipe, see page 205.) Excellent dippers can be made from broccoli, carrots, cauliflower, cherry tomatoes, green beans, red peppers, snow peas, turnips, and zucchini.
- Enlist your child's help in preparing the vegetables. If he helps wash and cut them up, he may be more interested in eating them.
- Make a delicious vegetable soup. Recipes for vegetable soups can be found in every cookbook.
- Green up your salads by adding spinach, romaine lettuce, or other dark greens. Additional vegetables you can add include cabbage, carrots, green peppers, and turnips. You can also add fruit such as apples, oranges, and pears to green salads. Choose the salad dressing carefully to avoid artificial colors, sugar, corn syrup, and partially hydrogenated oils.
- Encourage your child to drink a glass of tomato or V8 juice.
- Try a "one bite" policy. If your child takes one bite, he may take another and then another.

While your goal is to get your child to eat more fruits and vegetables, don't get into battles and power struggles over food. Keeping mealtime relaxed and happy is also important for your child's health.

Meat, Poultry, Fish, Dry Beans, Eggs, and Nuts

A healthy child's diet should also include two to three servings daily of lean meat, poultry, and fish; dry beans; eggs; and nuts. A serving is two to three ounces of cooked lean meat, poultry, or fish; a half cup of cooked dry beans; one egg; or two tablespoons of natural peanut butter (without sugar or partially hydrogenated fat). Lean meat, poultry, and fish supply complete protein, vitamins, and minerals. Cold-water fish, such as salmon, mackerel, and herring, are rich sources of the omega-3 essential fatty acids, which are crucial for nerve and brain function. Beans, including kidney, navy, pinto, soy, and red beans, are good sources of vitamins, minerals, fiber, and essential fatty acids. Nuts and seeds are delicious, ready-to-eat foods rich in essential fatty acids, iron, calcium, potassium, the B vitamins, vitamin E, complex carbohydrates, incomplete protein, and fiber. *A word of caution:* Do not give whole nuts or seeds to a child under the age of four. Young children can choke on these small, hard foods. Eggs are a superb source of many essential nutrients, including complete protein, minerals, and vitamins A, B_{12}, and D. Boiled or poached eggs are better for children than fried or scrambled eggs.

For some children, the more protein they have in their diet, the better they feel and act. As one mother commented, "My son needs a lot of protein to keep him on an even keel. We aim for three smaller meals and two to three high protein snacks. For example, his snacks often include a cup of plain yogurt or cottage cheese with fresh fruit, half a peanut butter sandwich on whole wheat with a dab of all-fruit preserves, a handful of nuts and a piece of fruit, or a cold chicken leg."

Milk, Yogurt, and Cheese

For the child who is not lactose intolerant and is not sensitive to milk, two to three servings of low-fat milk, yogurt, and cheese should be included in the diet every day. Milk, yogurt, and cheese provide complete protein, vitamins (especially vitamins A, B_{12}, and D, and riboflavin), and minerals (especially calcium). What counts as a serving? One cup of milk, one cup of yogurt, and one and a half ounces of natural cheese. Don't buy processed cheese that contains partially hydrogenated vegetable oil or food dye. Choose skim milk and nonfat yogurt whenever possible, since these are lower in fat than their regular counterparts. If your child dislikes milk and other milk products, or is sensitive to milk, he will need to take calcium supplements.

Fats, Oils, and Sweets

Fats, oils, and sweets are represented by the small tip of the Food Guide Pyramid because they should be eaten as little as possible. Sweets include soft drinks, candy, jam, jelly, syrup, and table sugar. Reduce the sugar in your child's diet. Restrict added sugar—including white sugar, brown sugar, raw sugar, fructose, maple syrup, honey, molasses, and corn syrup— to no more than six to ten teaspoons per day. Sweets supply calories and little else nutritionally. No *added sugar* is the goal for many kids with ADD or ADHD. The recipes beginning on page 193 of this book will give you ideas for how to replace sugary foods. Read the label on every food item you buy. If sugar or corn syrup is one of the first five ingredients, don't buy the item. You'll also find sugar listed on the new nutrition label, where it is reported in grams. Four grams of sugar equal one teaspoon. (For a more complete discussion of sweeteners in your child's diet, see "Choose Sweeteners Carefully," page 59.)

What about the fats and oils represented by the tip of the Food Guide Pyramid? Today, we often think of all fats as bad. However, there are "good" fats that your child must have for good health and normal brain function. Among sources of good fats are walnuts, beans (kidney, northern, black, soy, and navy), and fresh cold-water fish (tuna, salmon, and mackerel), which contain the omega-3 essential fatty acids. Pure, cold-pressed soybean and canola oils are good because they contain both the omega-3 and the omega-6 fatty acids. After opening a bottle of canola or soy oil, squeeze the contents of a vitamin-E capsule into the oil and gently disperse it by slowly turning the bottle upside-down several times without shaking it. Refrigerate the oil and encourage your child to consume about one to two tablespoons of it each day. You can help it go down easier by adding it to salad dressings and using it in your baked goods. Unfortunately, fatty acids are delicate molecules quickly destroyed by oxygen over time, so use up the oil as rapidly as possible. Frying also destroys the good molecules of fatty acids. (Olive oil doesn't provide essential fatty acids, but it's good for stovetop cooking because its nutrients are not destroyed by the oxygen in air.)

Reduce your child's consumption of all commercial solid shortenings made with hydrogenated fats. Also, limit his intake of foods containing partially hydrogenated vegetable oils, such as most margarines, crackers and baked goods, and some brands of mayonnaise. Using a small amount of butter is an alternative to using margarine. Whipped butter is even better because it doesn't contain as much saturated fat per teaspoon as regular butter. Commercial salad dressings are a problem. Many contain partially hydrogenated oil, corn sweetener, and sugar. They are often colored with artificial colors. A quadruple whammy! And fat-free salad dressings don't contain the "good" fats. Homemade salad dressings are the most nutritious choice—and not hard to prepare at all. (For easy recipes for French Dressing and Italian Dressing, see page 206.)

THE DIET OF AMERICAN CHILDREN

You probably are saying, "There's no way that my child meets the food pyramid guidelines. He doesn't even come close!" You have a lot of company. In a recent study, the food intake of more than 3,300 children and adolescents in the United States aged two to nineteen years was analyzed.[2] Here are the distressing high points:

- Only 1 percent of the children met all the recommendations of the Food Guide Pyramid.
- A total of 16 percent did not meet any of the recommendations.
- Only 30 percent met the recommendations for the fruit, grain, meat, and dairy groups.
- The total amount of fat the children consumed averaged 35 percent of their total calories.
- The added sugar (the sugar added to foods such as bread, cake, soft drinks, jam, and ice cream) averaged 15 percent of total calories.
- Nearly 50 percent of the children drank whole milk instead of low-fat milk.

The study concluded: "Children and teens in the United States follow eating patterns that do not meet national recommendations. Nutrition education and intervention are needed among US children."[3]

At first, your child and the rest of your family may rebel when you try to change their diets, but hang in there! It's hard to change patterns of eating overnight. I know, because I had to "clean up" my family's diet. I've also helped lots of other families make dietary changes.

Changing your family's diet doesn't have to be a complex process, however. You can simplify the process by making one change at a time. You don't have to make all the changes at once. In fact, your first step doesn't even have to involve your family, just you. When you go to the supermarket or prepare a meal, read labels. Learn what's in the different foods on your supermarket's shelves and in your pantry. Then, begin avoiding foods with artificial colors or flavors, or partially hydrogenated fat. Gradually decrease your use of sugary, high-fat foods, replacing them with seasonal fresh fruits. Replace snack foods with fruits and veggies, homemade popcorn, unsweetened cereal, and, occasionally, fat-free pretzels. If your child drinks soft drinks, replace them with uncolored sodas, such as Squirt, Sprite, and, if he can tolerate aspartame, Diet 7Up. After a while, replace the Diet 7Up with 100 percent pure fruit juice. Add omega-3 essential fatty acids to your family's diet by switching to pure, cold-pressed canola or soy oil.

Following is a basic meal plan to help you choose healthy foods for your family:

- Breakfast—lean meat, eggs, or low-fat yogurt; unsweetened fruit or 100 percent fruit juice; whole-grain bread or cereal; and low-fat milk
- Lunch—lean meat, fish, nut butter, cheese, or eggs; whole-grain bread, crackers, or rice cakes; raw veggies such as carrots or cherry tomatoes, or vegetable soup; fresh fruit; and milk or yogurt
- Snack—nut butter or cheese on whole-grain crackers; and veggies or fruit
- Dinner—lean meat, poultry, or fish (especially cold-water); brown rice, potato, or whole-grain bread; veggies such as sweet potato or broccoli, or vegetable soup; and fresh fruit
- Snack—nut butter on whole grain bread or crackers; and plain yogurt with fresh fruit

START THE DAY WITH A GOOD BREAKFAST

Do you remember when your mom would say, "Don't skip breakfast. It's the most important meal of the day"? Well, she was right! In the United States, breakfast consumption has declined steadily for the last twenty-five years. Of children aged eight and nine, 79 percent eat breakfast regularly, while only 58 percent of twelve- to thirteen-year-olds eat breakfast regularly.[4]

This is unfortunate, as the results of a recent study showed that the children who ate breakfast regularly demonstrated significantly higher reading and math scores, significantly lower reports of depression and anxiety, lower levels of hyperactivity, better school attendance, less tardiness, improved attention spans, fewer behavior problems, and fewer visits to the school nurse.[5] Conversely, other studies demonstrated that children who skipped breakfast had greater inattention problems and poorer scores on tests of cognitive tasks involving memory. In other words, children who are hungry have more problems paying attention and learning.

Breakfast should contribute about one-third of the day's calories and nutrients. A good breakfast enhances the quality of the daily diet and increases one's overall intake of fiber, vitamins, and minerals. Children who don't eat breakfast are often unable to make up for missed nutrients at later meals. If your child currently skips breakfast or has sugary, fat-laden, or nutrient-poor foods for breakfast, you must change his breakfast routine. (The table on pages 48–49 lists the content of sugar, partially hydrogenated oils, and artificial colors of some popular breakfast foods and drinks.) I know you already feel pressured in the morning trying to get your child ready for day care or school, but making time for breakfast will help the whole family. Enlist your family's help and support.

You may be tempted to serve your child cereal as a start to his day; however, buyer, beware! Many cereals, particularly those marketed toward children, are loaded with sugar and contain artificial colors and preservatives. (Recent well-designed studies have reported that many hyperactive children are often "turned on" by artificial colors.) The new nutritional labels provide valuable information on each box: a list of ingredients and the amount of sugars (natural and added) contained in a serving. The sugar information is listed as "grams per serving." Four grams equal 1 teaspoon. Choose cereals that are made from whole grains and contain no artificial colors and preservatives and less than one gram of sugar. The table on pages 50–51 gives the sugar and artificial-ingredient content of some popular cereals.

Try to avoid common breakfast meats like bacon and sausage. Bacon is a high-saturated fat food with little protein. It also contains sodium nitrite, which bothers some children. Most commercial sausage is high in fat and contains monosodium glutamate, which may bother some children. It's easy to make your own sausage from lean ground meat. See my recipe on page 196. Also avoid instant breakfast drinks. These are high in sugar. Again, a nutritious breakfast drink can easily be made at home. See my recipe on page 219.

Ingredients in Selected Breakfast Foods and Drinks That May Affect Your Child's ADD/ADHD

ITEM	AMOUNT OF SUGAR PER SERVING	ARTIFICIAL COLORS	PARTIALLY HYDROGENATED OILS	CHOCOLATE
Carnation French Vanilla Instant Breakfast	4¼ teaspoons	None	None	None
Carnation Classic Chocolate Malt Instant Breakfast	4¼ teaspoons	None	None	Yes
Nestlé Quik Chocolate	4½ teaspoons	None	None	Yes
Ovaltine Rich Chocolate	4½ teaspoons	Yellow #6, Red #40, Blue #1	None	Yes
Hershey's Chocolate Milk Mix	5¼ teaspoons	Caramel coloring, Red #40, Blue #1, Yellow #5	None	Yes

ITEM continued	AMOUNT OF SUGAR PER SERVING	ARTIFICIAL COLORS	PARTIALLY HYDROGENATED OILS	CHOCOLATE
Eggo Homestyle Waffles (2)	¾ teaspoon	Yellow #5 and #6	Yes	None
Strawberry Fruit Roll-Up	1¼ teaspoons	Red #40	Yes	None
Rice Krispies Treats	2 teaspoons	None	None	None
Jiffy Corn Muffins	2 teaspoons	None	Yes	None
Pillsbury Brown Sugar Cinnamon Toaster Strudel	2½ teaspoons	Yellow #5, Red #40	Yes	None
Nature Valley Oats 'n Honey Bars (2)	3 teaspoons	None	None	None
Hungry Jack Original Pancakes (3 4-inch pancakes)	3¼ teaspoons	None	Yes	None
Nutri-Grain Strawberry Cereal Bars	4 teaspoons	Red #40 and caramel colorings	Yes	None
Martha White Blueberry Muffins	3¼ teaspoons	Blue #2, Red #40, Yellow #5 and #6	Yes	None
SnackWell's Fat-Free Strawberry Cereal Bars	4 teaspoons	Red #40, Blue #1	None	None
Low-Fat Strawberry Pop Tart	4½ teaspoons	Red #40	Yes	None
Milk Chocolate Pop Tart	4½ teaspoons	Color added	Yes	Yes
Golden Griddle Syrup (4 tablespoons)	7½ teaspoons	Caramel coloring	None	None

Sugar and Artificial Ingredient Content of Selected Breakfast Cereals

CEREAL	AMOUNT OF SUGAR PER SERVING	ARTIFICIAL COLORS	PRESERVATIVES	CHOCOLATE
Cream of Rice	None	None	None	None
Puffed Rice	None	None	None	None
Cream of Wheat	None	None	None	None
Shredded Wheat	¼ teaspoon	None	BHT* (butylated hydroxytolvene)	None
Quaker Oatmeal	¼ teaspoon	None	None	None
Cheerios	¼ teaspoon	None	None	None
Post Toasties	½ teaspoon	None	BHT*	None
Corn Flakes	½ teaspoon	None	BHT*	None
Rice Chex	½ teaspoon	None	BHT	None
Rice Krispies	¾ teaspoon	None	BHT*	None
Corn Total	¾ teaspoon	None	BHT	None
Kix	¾ teaspoon	None	None	None
Wheaties	1 teaspoon	None	BHT	None
Grape Nut Flakes	1¼ teaspoons	None	None	None
Whole Grain Total	1¼ teaspoons	None	BHT	None
Life	1½ teaspoons	Yellow #5 and #6	BHT	None
Grape-Nuts	1¾ teaspoons	None	None	None
Cinnamon Toast Crunch	2½ teaspoons	Caramel coloring	BHT	None

*Present in packaging only.

CEREAL _continued_	AMOUNT OF SUGAR PER SERVING	ARTIFICIAL COLORS	PRESERVATIVES	CHOCOLATE
Cookie Crisp, chocolate chip	3 teaspoons	Blue #1, Red #40, Yellow #5 and #6	BHT	Yes
Cap'n Crunch	3 teaspoons	Yellow #5 and #6	BHT	None
Reese's Peanut Butter Puffs	3 teaspoons	Blue #5, Red #40, Blue #1, Caramel coloring	BHT	None
Frosted Flakes	3¼ teaspoons	None	BHT	None
Cocoa Pebbles	3¼ teaspoons	Caramel coloring	BHA (butylated hydroxyanisole)	Yes
Lucky Charms	3¼ teaspoons	Blue #1, Red #40, Yellow #5 and #6	None	None
Trix	3¼ teaspoons	Red #40, Yellow #6, Blue #1	None	None
Basic 4	3½ teaspoons	None	BHT	None
Cocoa Krispies	3½ teaspoons	None	BHT	Yes
Fruit Loops	3½ teaspoons	Blue #1, Blue #2, Red #40, Yellow #6	BHT	None
Apple Jacks	3½ teaspoons	Yellow #6, Red #40	BHT	None
Cocoa Puffs	3½ teaspoons	Caramel coloring	BHT	Yes
Natural Valley Oats and Honey	4¼ teaspoons	None	None	None
Raisin Bran	4½ teaspoons	None	None	None

Breakfast does not have to be complicated and time-consuming. The goal for breakfast should be to include both protein and complex carbohydrates. This combination will help your child feel better and pay attention all morning long. Here are some easy ideas.

- Eggs, one or two, preferably poached or boiled. Whole-grain bread with a little whipped butter and a dab of all-fruit preserves. Glass of low-fat milk.
- Small, lean broiled steak. Orange sections. Low-fat milk.
- Plain yogurt sweetened with fresh fruit. Whole-wheat pancakes with a little whipped butter and a dab of all-fruit preserves.
- Whole-grain cereal with low-fat milk. Leftover pork chop, chicken leg, roast beef.
- Whole-grain bread or rice cake with natural nut butter and a dab of all-fruit preserves. Low-fat milk.
- Grilled cheese sandwich made with whole-grain bread and real cheese, not processed cheese food. Piece of fruit. A glass of orange juice.
- Cottage cheese with fresh fruit. Whole-wheat toast with whipped butter. Unsweetened grapefruit juice.
- Cooked oatmeal with fresh fruit. Low-fat milk. Homemade sausage patty.
- Unprocessed nuts. A piece of fruit. Low-fat milk.

EATING WELL OUTSIDE THE HOME

Now that you are armed with the knowledge of what foods to buy and cook for your child at home, you need to know what choices to make when the menu is not entirely under your control. The following section will help you and your child make the proper selections when dining away from home.

Restaurants

You may be thinking, "We eat out a lot. How can we do this and still maintain a nutritionally sound diet?" The key is to make good choices. We occasionally eat at a nearby chain restaurant; however, we do our best to make good meal choices when eating there. For example, take a look at the following dinners:

Meal 1
Hamburger
French fries
Coke (12 ounces)
Apple pie

Meal 2
Vegetable soup
Grilled chicken tenderloin sandwich on 100 percent whole-wheat
   toast
Low-fat milk
Fruit cup

What are the nutritional differences between these two meals? Meal 1 has about 400 more calories than Meal 2. Meal 1 also has three times the total fat and saturated fat, half the fiber, one-third the magnesium, far less vitamin A, one-fourth the calcium, and one-half the vitamin C. Zinc and iron levels in the two meals are about the same. So take a minute to read the menus at your favorite restaurant and choose foods carefully. All family members should make an effort to choose foods wisely.

Choosing nutritious meals is harder at fast-food restaurants. Here are some suggestions. Choose grilled chicken instead of hamburgers, baked potato instead of French fries, and milk or 100 percent fruit juice instead of soda. From the salad bar, choose unsweetened fresh fruit or canned fruit in its own juice, fresh vegetables, and salad with vinegar and oil dressing instead of sweet, artificially colored salad dressing. You also might choose cottage cheese or unsweetened applesauce. Skip the gelatin "salads."

School Lunches

In some schools it's "cool" to bring your lunch and in others it's not. Dealing with lunches the school provides is often a discouraging task. If your child really wants to eat the school lunch, perhaps you can compromise on the frequency. Most school districts provide menus in advance so you can choose days that are more nutritional than others. For example, here are three unacceptable lunches provided this month by my school district:

- Sausage patties
- French toast sticks with maple syrup
- Cinnamon applesauce
- Fruit punch, milk

- Cheeseburger
- Tater sticks
- Fruit cocktail
- Strawberry Fruit Roll-Up
- Milk

- Pepperoni Pizza Pocket
- Pineapple canned in heavy syrup
- Apple juice, milk
- Hostess Twinkie

Those lunches are high in sugar and fat. They also may contain artificial colors. Here are three other lunches, offered this month, that are more nutritious. They are lower in fat and sugars and probably don't contain artificial colors.

- Roast turkey
- Mashed potatoes/gravy
- Peaches
- Milk

- Taco snack
- Cheesy broccoli
- Pineapple tidbits
- Milk

- Taco salad (taco meat, lettuce, cheese, taco shell)
- Peaches canned in juice
- Milk

If your child brings his lunch from home, here are some tips:

- Younger children enjoy carrying a lunch box filled with a variety of good foods. Most older children prefer to "brown-bag it" with a sandwich, veggies, and a piece of fruit.
- Enlist your child's help in packing the lunch box or bag lunch. If your child helps choose and prepare the foods, he's more likely to eat them.
- If milk is tolerated, have your child buy low-fat white milk instead of chocolate milk.
- To save time in the morning prepare as much of the lunch as possible the night before. Sandwich spreads can be made the night before. Sliced meat or cheese (real cheese, not "cheese food" or "cheese product") sandwiches can be made at night and wrapped up tightly in waxed paper. Wrap lettuce leaves separately so they don't wilt. Then your child can add the lettuce right before he eats the sandwich.
- If your child is sensitive to wheat, try wrapping his favorite sandwich spread in cabbage, spinach, or romaine lettuce leaves. Insert a toothpick to hold the "sandwich" together. Or stuff green peppers or potato skins with sandwich spread.
- Send a couple of spoonfuls of a cheese ball (made from real cheese, not "cheese food" or "cheese product"). Include a plastic knife and whole-grain crackers or celery.
- Choose natural peanut butter made from just peanuts and salt

(no sugar or hydrogenated vegetable oils). Spread on whole-wheat bread or crackers or rice cakes. Top with a dab of all-fruit preserves (no sugar added). You can find other nut and seed butters at your health-food store.

- Slice an apple in half and remove the core. Spread with peanut butter and top with a few raisins or banana slices. Put halves back together and wrap in waxed paper.

- Spread pizza sauce on toasted whole-wheat English muffins. Top with cheese. Place under broiler until cheese melts. Refrigerate. Wrap in waxed paper.

- Hot dishes like homemade macaroni and cheese, stew, chili, or homemade soup may be packed in a wide-mouth thermos. Include whole-grain crackers and necessary utensils.

- Choose refried beans and whole-wheat pita pockets or taco shells. Pack filling separately from pockets or shells.

- Pack cold foods like unsweetened applesauce, unsweetened fruit salad, cottage cheese and homemade gelatin salads in wide-mouth thermos.

- Instead of packing a sandwich, include a piece of meat (like baked chicken), a slice of meatloaf, a couple of homemade meatballs, or deviled eggs. Include a piece of whole-grain bread spread lightly with whipped butter and a dab of all-fruit (no sugar added) preserves.

- Include a whole piece of fruit—a banana, apple, pear, peach, plum, or grapes.

- Unprocessed nuts may be included. Also a small bag of homemade air-popped or microwaved popcorn (made from only popcorn kernels and salt) make good snacks.

- A few pieces of unsweetened dried fruits may be included if tolerated.

- Include carrots, cherry tomatoes, or other cut-up vegetables and natural peanut butter or a vegetable dip.

- Your child may enjoy a small can of 100 percent unsweetened fruit juice.

In his twenty-five years of practicing pediatrics, William Sears, M.D., author of *The A.D.D. Book*, has noted that healthier children eat healthier diets:

> *Mothers who consistently do not allow any unhealthy food to pollute the bodies of their children have healthier children. These children have fewer office visits and fewer colds, and when they come for periodic checkups, they seem more settled and better behaved. These "pure children" seem to get tagged with fewer labels, such as "A.D.D." or "learning disability." And even when these children do warrant such tags, they seem to cope better with their behavioral and learning differences, which also seem less severe.[6]*

If your child is a "junk-food addict," improve his diet. If he is to enjoy good physical and mental health, he must eat good, nutritious food from a variety of sources. Improving your family's diet probably won't be easy. But a nutritionally sound diet will benefit all family members for a lifetime. As one mother commented in *Help for the Hyperactive Child*, by William Crook, M.D.: "Even though you're overwhelmed, don't be discouraged. Keep it simple. Don't let remarks from a friend, neighbor or relative bother you. You can't learn everything at once. Start with basic meats, vegetables, fruits and whole grains. These products are easy to prepare once you've set up your kitchen. Doing it this way is easier than shopping for all of the other kinds of confusing products. If you learn on a gradual basis to feed your family with simple foods, things get much less confusing. Don't beat yourself to death emotionally if you don't do things perfectly."[7]

Saul Pilar, M.D., had these words of wisdom for parents:

> *You want the best school, the best teachers, the best books, the best clothes, the best sports activities for your child. How about your child's nutrition? Are you going to give him a better chance or are you going to give him another handicap—suboptimal nutrition? If you want your child to have A + marks, don't give him a C − diet, please.[8]*

The same principles apply to adults who have ADD or ADHD. Some adults can greatly improve their inattention and behavior by improving their diet. Here's what forty-year-old David, who had been diagnosed by his psychologist as having ADD, had to say:

> *Since I started eliminating the junk in my diet, I am beginning to feel normal again. In fact, I feel like a different person. My attention at work and home have greatly improved. Caffeine in Coke and coffee has been a real problem for me. Also artificial sweeteners, sugar, artificial colors and preservatives in Coke, gum and candy. I was really addicted to these "foods." I've struggled to give up these foods, but the results are worth all the effort.*

Remember, you don't have to change all of your family's meals at once. Concentrate on one meal at a time. Work on that one meal for as long as necessary—one day, one week, or one month. You'll know you have succeeded when your child asks you for an apple as a snack instead of the usual apple toaster pastry!

WAY 2.
CHOOSE
SWEETENERS
CAREFULLY

What's the story with sugar? The studies that so far have been done on sugar have had mixed results. In some, a number of the children in the study reacted to sugar, and in others, none of the children had reactions.[1] Some of the studies were flawed because they used aspartame, chocolate, milk, citrus, or wheat to disguise the sugar. These foods and food additives turn some children on by themselves. Many parents don't care what any of the studies have said, however. They know beyond a shadow of a doubt that sugar changes their children from a Dr. Jekyll to a Mr. Hyde. Parents really do know best. Trust your instincts.

To help determine how your child is affected by sugar, answer yes or no to the following questions:

1. Does your child consume one or more glasses of soft drinks each day?
2. Does your child drink fruit punch rather than 100 percent unsweetened fruit juice?

3. Does your child eat a lot of cookies, candy, and sugary desserts?
4. Does your child start the day with highly sugared cereal?
5. Does your child crave sugar? Is he a "sugarholic"?
6. Has your child ever stolen candy or money to buy candy?
7. Do your child's behavior problems worsen around the holidays?
8. Does your child suffer repeated ear infections and take many rounds of antibiotics?

If you answered no to the above questions, congratulations! You can skip to the next chapter. However, if you answered yes to one or more of the questions, this chapter will show you some ways in which you can decrease the sugar in your child's diet.

SUGAR AND OTHER NATURAL SWEETENERS

You read in the last chapter how much sugar is found in popular children's cereals. You may also be surprised by how much sugar is added to children's other favorite foods. The table on page 61 gives examples.

Sugar is loaded with "naked calories." It has no fiber, complex carbohydrates, vitamins, or minerals. Studies show that the average American adult consumes more than 120 pounds of refined sugar a year. Many American children take in that much or more. That amount—120 pounds—really is amazing. Picture your shopping cart loaded with more than twenty five-pound bags of sugar! As one researcher commented, "High sucrose diets, with sucrose ranging from 25 to 60 percent of caloric intake, may be displacing essential minerals, vitamins, and amino acids necessary for brain function. This would explain why most controlled, low-dose, short-duration, double-blind studies fail to find a relation between sucrose and behavior, despite widespread public belief to the contrary."[2]

Then there is the hidden sugar in foods ranging from ketchup to salad dressing to canned peas. You must read labels carefully. The following are all names for sugar: brown sugar, cane sugar, confectioners' sugar, raw sugar, turbinado sugar, molasses, natural sweetener, sucrose. Natural sweeteners such as corn syrup, dextrose, fructose, and glucose are also sugars

Sugar Content of Favorite Foods

FOOD	SERVING SIZE	ADDED SUGAR
Fruit drink	12 ounces	12 teaspoons
Chocolate shake	10 ounces	9 teaspoons
Cola drink	12 ounces	9 teaspoons
Fruit yogurt	1 cup	7 teaspoons
Frosted cake	¹⁄₁₆ of cake	6 teaspoons
Fruit pie	⅙ of pie	6 teaspoons
Fruit, canned in heavy syrup	½ cup	4 teaspoons
Gelatin	½ cup	4 teaspoons
Chocolate bar	1 ounce	3 teaspoons
Chocolate milk	1 cup	3 teaspoons
Fruit, canned in juice	½ cup	0
Plain yogurt	1 cup	0

and loaded with empty calories. Honey and maple syrup too should be avoided as they are liquid sugars with few essential nutrients.

Sugar seems to be addictive for some children. One hyperactive child would lick his fingers as he passed the sugar canister, dip his wet fingers into the sugar, and then lick them clean. He'd figured out how to get his fix! Another perceptive child would scream, "I need sugar *now*!" If your child is a sugarholic, you may need to decrease his sugar intake slowly over a period of a few weeks rather than abruptly removing it from his diet. As one mother explained:

Our three-year-old son would waken in the middle of the night screaming for 7Up. To quiet him, we would give him a few ounces. Embarrassed, I finally brought this problem up with our nutritionally oriented doctor. His recommendation was to give Tommy 2 ounces of sugary 7Up mixed with 2 ounces of sugar-free 7Up [which was artificially sweetened with saccharin]. Then we gradually shifted to the sugar-free 7Up and finally to 100 percent fruit juices. By then, Tommy had stopped waking in the middle of the night

and slept peacefully. His days were much calmer. I can't believe how foolish
we were to have given him soft drinks in the first place.

You may need to reduce the sugar in your house gradually. Don't have a big discussion about it. Instead, just do it. For example, in place of cookies with icing, buy cookie wafers. Stop buying candy. Replace fruit drinks with 100 percent pure fruit juices. Replace sugary treats with healthy snacks and foods.

See what works best for your child. Try a no-sugar diet for a couple of weeks. Read all labels carefully. Note that your child's symptoms may be worse during the first few days. Then give your child sugar for a few days and observe his behavior. Is he more hyperactive? Is he depressed? Does he complain of any physical symptoms, such as muscle aches, headache, or runny nose? If he is better on the sugar-free diet and worse when sugar is added back to his diet, then you have identified one of the pieces of your child's hyperactivity puzzle. Even if your child does not seem to react to sugar, maintain a low-sugar diet so that he'll have room for nutritious foods.

OTHER SWEETENERS

If sugar is a no-no, what can you use instead? The first choice is whole fruit, filled with natural sweetness to satisfy a child's desire for sweets. You can also use concentrated 100 percent apple, grape, pineapple, or orange juice to flavor foods. Following are some other alternatives. You'll have to decide what works best for your child.

Saccharin

Saccharin is 300 times sweeter than table sugar. Synthesized from coal tar, it was discovered by accident in 1879. By the turn of the century, it was used in place of sugar in some canned vegetables and beverages. Over the years, the use of saccharin has increased. However, in 1977, experiments showed that large amounts of saccharin could produce bladder tumors in rodents. The Food and Drug Administration (FDA) therefore moved to ban saccharin. The public outcry was so loud, Congress passed specific legislation to delay the ban. This delay was extended several times. Until recently, every product that contains saccharin has been required to carry the following warning: "Use of this product may be hazardous to your health. This product contains saccharin which has been determined to cause cancer in laboratory animals." More recent studies in which large doses of saccharin were given to mice, hamsters, and monkeys have shown no cancer-causing effects. Also, studies have not shown an increased risk for bladder cancer in the human population. There are no studies to suggest that saccharin does or doesn't cause behavior changes in children. Nonetheless, pregnant women and young children should avoid saccharin.

If you decide to use saccharin, use it sparingly—a packet or so a day. Fasweet, Superose, Sweeta, and Sweet'n Low are all sweeteners containing saccharin that you can find at your grocery store. You can sweeten hot beverages and bake with saccharin, since it is not affected by heat. Your child may or may not dislike the aftertaste of saccharin.

Cyclamate

Cyclamate was discovered in 1937—accidentally, the same as saccharin. Cyclamate is thirty times sweeter than sugar. It has a pleasant taste and acts as a flavor enhancer. It's used as a tabletop sweetener and in diet beverages and other low-calorie foods. It remains stable at high and low temperatures and has a long shelf life. It can be used in cooking and baking.

Cyclamate was used widely in the United States in the 1950s and 1960s. However, in 1969, experiments suggested that it could cause bladder cancer in mice and rats. The FDA therefore banned the sweetener in 1970, and today the ban remains in effect in the United States. However, cyclamate is used widely in forty other countries, including Canada. The effect of cyclamate on the behavior of children with ADD has not been studied. If you have access to this sweetener, use it sparingly and cautiously.

Aspartame

Like saccharin and cyclamate, aspartame was discovered accidentally. It is comprised of two amino acids (phenylalanine and aspartate) joined together, and is 200 times sweeter than sugar. It is widely found in processed foods—ice cream, diet soft drinks, gelatin desserts, puddings, and breakfast cereals—and as a tabletop sweetener sold under the brand names Equal, Natra Taste, and NutraSweet. Unlike saccharin, aspartame has no aftertaste and acts like a flavor enhancer. Also unlike saccharin, aspartame cannot be used for baking because prolonged heat breaks it down, causing its sweet taste to be lost. However, you can get around this in many recipes by adding the aspartame after the cooking stage. For example, if you are making Blueberry Syrup (see page 203), cook the blueberries in the water until soft, then remove the mixture from the heat and stir in the aspartame.

Although aspartame is one of the most highly studied food additives ever approved for use in the United States, great controversies remain over its safety. Some scientists have worried that using aspartame in great amounts could raise the amount of phenylalanine and aspartate in the blood to potentially harmful levels. High blood levels of phenylalanine are dangerous for people with the genetic disorder phenylketonuria (PKU), which severely affects the central nervous system. Therefore, all products containing aspartame must carry the warning "Phenylketonurics: Contains Phenylalanine." Another concern is that aspartame raises blood-methanol levels. However, methanol is a natural constituent of the diet and is found in canned fruit and vegetable juices in levels comparable to those in a liter of aspartame-sweetened soft drink.

A number of troubling symptoms have been reported by aspartame users. These include headaches, insomnia, dizziness, fatigue, anxiety, irritability, and depression. There have been concerns that aspartame can be toxic to the central nervous system, especially in children. Some parents have reported that their children showed increased hyperactivity following ingestion of aspartame. One child was studied very carefully by renowned researcher C. K. Conners, Ph.D., who included among his methods a double-blind challenge. He reports what this four-year-old child's mother experienced when the boy drank red diet Kool-Aid:

> *She told me that during the summer Jamie drank diet Kool-Aid for about three weeks, usually about three glasses a day. Over this period of time she noticed that he became increasingly erratic, with gradually escalating levels*

of frustration, anger, and emotionality. He easily burst into tears, was very irritable, and had violent, unprovoked, angry outbursts. Eventually, he had an episode when he became so hyperactive that he had to be sent to his room, whereupon he proceeded to throw himself against a wall, knocking himself to the floor, repeating this behavior until restrained. He was totally out of control in a way she had not seen before.[3]

Jamie's doctor recommended that the boy no longer be given diet Kool-Aid, and the boy's behavior returned to normal. When Jamie drank diet red Kool-Aid again ten days later, he became even more violent and complained of a severe headache. Interestingly, Jamie had no problems with red Kool-Aid made with sugar. It was only diet red Kool-Aid made with aspartame that dramatically changed his behavior.

Other studies have looked at the effects of sugar and aspartame on the behavior and cognitive performance of children. One study targeted pre-schoolers from three to five years old and school-aged children from six to ten years old. It compared the effects of a diet high in sucrose, a diet high in aspartame, and a diet high in saccharin. The researchers concluded: "Even when intake exceeds typical dietary levels, neither dietary sucrose nor aspartame affects children's behavior or cognitive function."[4]

So where does this leave you, the confused parent? Try an aspartame-free diet for a couple of weeks. Is your child better? When you reintroduce aspartame, does he become worse? If your answer is yes to both questions, avoid aspartame. However, if your answer is no, you can use aspartame, but do so in very low amounts, such as a packet or two a day, if at all.

Acelsulfame-K

Acelsulfame-K is another artificial sweetener that is manmade. It is 200 times sweeter than sugar. Unlike aspartame, acelsulfame does not break down when heated, so it can be used in baked goods. It is not metabolized by the body and is excreted unchanged in the urine.

Acelsulfame-K has been approved for use in chewing gum, powdered drink mixes, and gelatins, and as a tabletop sweetener. It is currently sold under the brand name of Sweet One. However, concerns have been raised about acelsulfame's safety, and some scientists have called for further testing for toxicity and cancer-causing properties. Right now, it is better to limit your use of acelsulfame to small amounts.

Sucralose

Sucralose is a new artificial sweetener that was approved for use in United States in 1998. It was discovered in 1976 and has undergone more than a hundred scientific studies. Sucralose is the only artificial sweetener made from sugar. Three chlorine atoms are substituted for sugar's three hydrogen-oxygen groups. (Chlorine in this form is not harmful—after all, salt, or sodium chloride, contains a chlorine atom.) It's about 600 times sweeter than sugar and has no calories. It has no unpleasant aftertaste. It withstands high heat and low pH (acidity) very well, and does not break down over time. It can be used in beverages, ice cream, chewing gum, baked goods, desserts, dairy products, syrups, condiments, and processed fruits, and functions well as a tabletop sweetener.

Sucralose is not metabolized by the body. Instead, it passes through the body unchanged and is eliminated. Extensive studies have reported that sucralose does not cause cancer or neurological problems. It has also been reported to be safe for pregnant women, breast-feeding mothers, and children.

Sucralose, marketed under the brand name of Splenda, is not yet widely available in the United States. Only time will tell whether sucralose has any side effects that have not been uncovered by all the scientific studies. Until more is known, use sucralose cautiously and in small amounts.

Sorbitol

Sorbitol is a sugar-alcohol. Sugar-alcohol occurs widely in nature, but sorbitol is usually produced commercially from glucose. Sorbitol is about 60 percent as sweet as sugar, with one-third the calories. It has a sweet, cool, and pleasant taste, with no aftertaste. Sorbitol is very stable and can withstand high temperatures. It cannot be metabolized by the bacteria in the mouth, so it does not promote tooth decay.

Sorbitol is found in many food products, including chewing gum, candy, frozen desserts, cookies, cakes, icings, and fillings. It is also found in toothpaste and mouthwash. It does not seem to be sold as a tabletop sweetener. Products from which consumers are likely to ingest a high level of sorbitol must carry the warning "Excess consumption may have a laxative effect." So sorbitol may cause your child to have gas and diarrhea.

Sorbitol is absorbed more slowly than sugar, which may be an advantage for hyperactive kids who react to sugar. It is possible to find white peppermint candies sweetened with sorbitol. If tolerated, one or two of these might be used for special occasions. You'll have to see what works best for your child.

Stevia

Stevia is a natural sweetener that comes from an herb that has been growing in Latin America for centuries. It is anywhere from 30 to 300 times sweeter than sugar and is used throughout the world as a noncaloric sweetener. In the United States, the FDA has approved its use as a dietary supplement.

Stevia can be used in hot and cold beverages, and also in baked goods. It's expensive, but a pinch will sweeten a glass of your favorite beverage. One teaspoon has the sweetening power of about two to four cups of sugar.

A downside of stevia is that it often has an unpleasant aftertaste. Therefore, some people use stevia only in foods that have strong flavors. Another downside is that stevia may cause infertility in women. However, because it is sold in the United States as a food supplement, it does not have to submit to the rigorous safety testing required by the FDA to verify this.

•

Keeping sugar out of a young child's diet can be difficult, especially when there is so much confusion surrounding the use of sugar substitutes. Perhaps one solution to the problem is to use several different kinds in small amounts, each on a different day. This approach reduces your child's exposure to any one sweetener.

WAY 3.
TRACK DOWN
HIDDEN FOOD
ALLERGIES

At some point you may have said to your doctor, "You know, every time my child eats chocolate or red dye, his behavior worsens—he becomes irritable and hyperactive, and can't pay attention." And your doctor probably replied, "Oh, no. There's no connection. The idea that specific foods or additives can alter behavior was just a fad in the 1970s that's been disproved. Diet has nothing to do with ADHD." And it's true that most early studies did not show a connection except in a small group of children. However, better-designed studies published in first-rate medical journals in the late 1980s and early 1990s have reported that food sensitivities are a major cause of ADHD symptoms in many children (more than 70 percent). Excellent studies have also shown that food sensitivities are common causes of headaches (including migraines), seizures, ear infections, and bed-wetting in children. (For more information on these fascinating studies, see Appendix A, "Scientific Studies for You and Your Doctor.")

Some allergies, including asthma, hay fever, eczema, and hives, are obvious. Respiratory allergies are easy to recognize when your child sneezes, coughs, or wheezes while playing with the cat, raking leaves, eating a picnic lunch during ragweed season, or rummaging around a dusty, moldy attic. If your child swells, itches, and breaks out in hives when he eats lobster, strawberries, or peanuts, he has an obvious food allergy.

In contrast, "hidden" food allergies aren't discovered unless they're specifically sought. These are usually caused by foods that are eaten every day, including chocolate, milk, eggs, wheat, rye, corn, citrus, legumes, and sugar. Other commonly eaten foods may also cause reactions. Unfortunately, different children have different sensitivities, so there is no single diet that works for everyone. Food allergies develop slowly, so the relationship between food and behavior often is not clear. Unlike obvious allergies, which are mediated by immunoglobulin E (IgE), hidden food-induced reactions are not. Therefore, allergy scratch tests are usually negative. Other kinds of lab tests are still under study but show promise.

To help determine if your child has hidden food allergies, answer yes or no to the following questions:

1. Does your child appear pale?
2. Does your child have dark shadows or bags under his eyes?
3. Does your child have a chronically stuffy nose?
4. Does your child sniff, snort, clear his throat, or push his nose up?
5. Does your child have recurrent ear infections or tubes in his ears?
6. Does your child have frequent stomachaches for which your doctor has ruled out obvious causes?
7. Does your child frequently have pain in his legs or other muscles or joints?
8. Does your child have persistent colds, bronchitis, asthma, or sinus?
9. Does your child have recurrent headaches?
10. Does your child wet the bed?
11. Does your child get pink or red cheeks or ears after eating certain foods?
12. Does your child show irritability and nervousness?
13. Does your child appear "spaced out"?

14. Does your child have trouble paying attention?
15. Does your child act better if he skips a meal?
16. Does your child feel and act worse after eating? Does his nose suddenly become stuffy?
17. Does your child have periods of fatigue, drowsiness, weakness, malaise, or depression?
18. Is your child a picky eater?
19. Does your child crave certain foods?
20. Does your child frequently get mouth ulcers or canker sores? Does his mouth look like a map (geographic tongue)? Does he have bad breath?
21. Does your child have relatives (parents, grandparents, or siblings) with allergies?
22. Does your child have obvious allergies himself?

If you answered no to the above questions, consider yourself fortunate. It's not easy to live without allergies in today's sprayed-, processed-, engineered-food world. However, if you answered yes to any of the questions, this chapter will show you how to track down hidden food allergies in your child.

THE COMMON FOODS ELIMINATION DIET

The best way to track down hidden food allergies in both children and adults is the Common Foods Elimination Diet. On this diet, the foods that are eaten most often are avoided. If your child is allergic to the foods he's avoiding, his symptoms will improve or disappear. The symptoms will return when he eats the foods again.

The Common Foods Elimination Diet is designed for the "average" child who lives in the United States, Canada, the British Isles, Australia, or New Zealand. Every day, these children consume cow's milk; wheat; corn; eggs; soy, peanuts, peas, beans, or other legumes; citrus; chocolate; cane or beet sugar; or food colorings, dyes, or additives. In the last ten years, these particular foods have been identified as the most common causes of ADHD in several scientific studies. If your child regularly eats or craves any of these foods or foods containing them, be suspicious.

In addition, for some foods, you should be suspicious for a few additional reasons. For example, you should be suspicious of milk if your child consumed a milk-based formula as a baby and had trouble with colic, frequent spitting up, skin rashes, eczema, or frequent ear infections. Milk might also be a problem for your child if any of his blood relatives avoid milk because it makes them sick. Does your child either crave or hate milk, cheese, yogurt, ice cream, or creamy foods? Does your child drink more than 16 ounces of milk a day?

In addition to craving sugar, does your child crave sugary soft drinks? Has he ever stolen candy or money to buy candy? Does he ever eat sugar just by itself? Does he get up in the middle of the night to eat something sugary?

Does your child's behavior worsen over the holidays, when artificially colored and flavored candies and foods are readily available? Does his behavior worsen at any time of the year when he eats these "treats"? If yes, food colorings, dyes, or additives may be a problem.

With the Common Foods Elimination Diet, you'll be able to determine which of these foods and others are a problem for your child. The diet consists of two parts. First, you will eliminate a number of your child's usual foods to see if his symptoms improve or disappear. Then, after five to ten days, when your child shows convincing improvement, give him the eliminated foods again, one at a time, to see which ones cause the symptoms. See Appendix B, "Jimmy's Common Foods Elimination Diet and Diary," to see how one child's symptoms were recorded. It will also give you some ideas for menus.

Keep a record of your child's symptoms in a notebook. (For a sample form to use, see Appendix B.) Start the diary three days before beginning the diet. Continue keeping it while your child is on the elimination portion of the diet and then while he's eating the eliminated foods again. You may find it helpful to grade your child's symptoms. For example, use 0 for no symptoms, 1 for mild symptoms, 2 for moderate symptoms, and 3 for severe symptoms.

During the first two to four days of the diet, your child is apt to feel irritable, hungry, and more hyperactive. He may develop a headache or leg cramps. He may have dark circles under his eyes. He may hate the diet, but hang in there! The stakes are high. If the foods he's avoiding are the cause of his symptoms, he'll usually feel better by the fourth, fifth, or sixth day of the diet. Almost always, he'll be improved by the tenth day.

After you're certain that your child is feeling and behaving better, and his improvement has lasted for at least two days, begin adding foods back to his diet, one at a time. If he's allergic to one or more of the eliminated foods, he'll usually develop a headache, stuffy nose, behavior problems, or other symptoms when he eats the food again. These symptoms will usually appear within a few minutes to a few hours. However, sometimes you may not notice symptoms until the next day.

Foods to Avoid on the Common Foods Elimination Diet

To prepare for the Common Foods Elimination Diet you'll want to read labels carefully. Here are some pointers.

Chocolate, Cocoa, and Cola   Chocolate, cocoa, cola, and coffee all belong to the same food family, so a sensitivity to one may mean a sensitivity to other family members. These foods can be very addictive so you may want to decrease the amount your child is consuming over a week or two, then remove these foods totally from your child's diet. If you're eating away from home, be sure to ask about hidden ingredients. I once ate chili that contained a "secret" ingredient. It turned out to be cocoa!

Cane and Beet Sugar   Labels on sugar bags or boxes may not state whether the sugar is cane or beet. Which one is used will depend on where you live and the current price of each sugar. Occasionally, a child will be sensitive to one sugar but not the other. But neither sugar should be encouraged. If your child is a sugar addict, review Way 2, on sweeteners. Reduce his sugar intake gradually before you start the elimination diet.

The following ingredients mean cane or beet sugar may be present:

Sucrose
Brown sugar
Natural sweetener
Molasses
Confectioners' sugar
Raw sugar
Turbinado sugar
Cane

Artificial Colorings   Artificial colorings are found in many prepared foods such as cake mixes, butter, cheese, ice cream, crackers, soups, hot dogs, pastries, and jams. Read labels on foods, cosmetics, and over-the-counter drugs carefully. Ask your pharmacist or doctor if a prescribed medicine contains dyes and whether or not there is a white replacement. Look for the following on product labels: U.S. certified colors, Yellow #5, Yellow #6, Red #3, Red #40, Blue #1, Blue #2, Green #3, any color that has a number, artificial colors added, FD & C colors (a label of only "D & C" means that the color cannot be used in foods, just in drugs and cosmetics—definitely avoid any product labeled this way), and tartrazine.

If the label says "Natural color added," the food may be okay. Natural colors include annatto, carmine (cochineal extract), and beta-carotene. However, severe obvious allergic reactions, including sneezing, asthma, and shock, have occurred occasionally after sensitive people consumed annatto or carmine.

Milk   Cow's milk is the most common food allergen in the United States. On the Common Foods Elimination Diet, avoid cow's milk and goat's milk in all forms. Milk is often found in breads, soups, margarines, powdered artificial sweeteners, so-called nondairy creamers, cereals, luncheon meats, vegetables with butter or milk sauces, and dessert mixes, to name just a few. When reading labels, watch out for the following terms, which mean milk:

Nonfat dried milk solids
Evaporated milk

Condensed milk

Lactose

Whey

Cream

Cheese

Butter

Margarine

Casein

Calcium caseinate

Sodium caseinate

Lactalbumin

Curds

Yogurt

Lactate

Your child can survive quite well without milk for the duration of the Common Foods Elimination Diet. Although milk supplies protein, phosphorus, and vitamins A, D, and B_{12} these nutrients are available elsewhere. If you find that your child is sensitive to milk, you'll want to supplement his diet with calcium, which is essential for building strong bones and teeth.

Corn Corn rivals milk for the top spot on the list of allergy-causing foods. Corn is widely used in many forms and is commonly found in table salt, confectioners' sugar, chewing gum, baking powder, margarine, ketchup, pickles, cereals, sweetened fruit juices, fruits packed in syrup, hot dogs, luncheon meats, mixed vegetables, soups, and vitamins. Corn may also be found in nonfood items such as toothpaste, aspirin, many medications, cough syrup, stamps, gummed labels, envelopes, and paper cups— just to name a few! Some of the vitamin C used in supplements is derived from corn. The following ingredients suggest corn may be present:

Syrup

Dextrose

Cornstarch

Dextrine
Starch
Glucose
Hominy
Fructose
Grits
Shortening
Sugar
Vegetable oil
Corn sweeteners
Maize
Sweeteners
Malt

For a corn elimination diet, you'll want to find a corn-free baking powder. You will also need to use pure corn-free vegetable oil, such as canola oil, and a milk-free, corn-free margarine.

Wheat and Rye   Some children are sensitive to all grains (wheat, rye, oats, barley, rice), but sometimes if one grain isn't tolerated others can be. On this diet, you should avoid wheat, barley, and rye, which are closely related. Your child may eat oats, rice, and nongrain substitutes (see Part 3). Remember, most commercial rye, potato, and oat breads all contain wheat flour. When reading labels, watch for the following ingredients:

Flour
Durum flour
Wheat flour
Semolina
Whole-wheat flour
Gluten flour
Wheat germ
Enriched flour

Graham flour
Monosodium glutamate (MSG)
Bran
Spelt

Eggs   Avoid both egg whites and egg yolks on the Common Foods Elimination Diet. Eggs are commonly found in baked goods, noodles, root beer, some breads, mayonnaise, tartar sauce, ice cream, and some egg-substitute products. They are also found in live vaccines for polio, mumps, and measles. Some terms indicating the presence of eggs in a product are:

Vitellin
Albumin
Powdered eggs
Globulin
Egg whites
Dried eggs
Ovomucin
Egg yolks
Whole eggs

Citrus Fruits   Fruits to avoid on this diet are oranges, grapefruits, ugli fruit, lemons, limes, kumquats, and tangerines. You do not need to avoid citric acid. Test those citrus fruits your child eats frequently. Avoid the others during the elimination diet.

If your child is sensitive to all citrus fruits, you will want to be sure he is getting enough vitamin C in his diet. Other good food sources of vitamin C are cantaloupe, tomato, guava, mango, papaya, broccoli, Brussels sprouts, and green peppers. Your child may need to take vitamin C tablets as discussed in Way 5.

Legumes   Peas, green beans, carob, peanuts, and soybeans are all related. Soy is particularly difficult to avoid as it is found everywhere—in shortening, baked goods, vitamins, breads, mayonnaise, salad dressings, and infant formulas. Lecithin and food extenders are soy derivatives. Test those legumes your child eats frequently. Avoid the other legumes during the elimination diet.

•

Your child is unique, and if he eats bananas, apples, potatoes, rice, beef, chicken, or other favorite foods every day, you'll need to modify these instructions to eliminate the foods that are most apt to be causing his symptoms.

After your child has completed the elimination part of his diet, add the following foods to his diet—one food per day. Start with those foods you least suspect. Make sure you add the foods in pure form. Here are suggestions.

Egg: Hard-boiled or scrambled in pure safflower, sunflower, or canola oil.

Citrus: Fresh orange sections.

Milk: Use pure milk.

Wheat: Use Cream of Wheat or Shredded Wheat.

Food coloring: Buy a set of McCormick's or French's dyes and colors. Put a half teaspoon of each color in a glass. Add a teaspoon of that mixture to a glass of water.

Chocolate: Use Baker's cooking chocolate or Hershey's cocoa powder. You can sweeten it with liquid saccharin.

Corn: Use fresh corn on the cob.

Sugar: Use plain cane sugar.

Peanuts: Use fresh peanuts roasted in the shell or unprocessed peanut butter. *Do not* test peanuts if your child has ever had a bad reaction to them.

Following the Common Foods Elimination Diet is not at all easy. It takes a lot of planning and determination. Here are some other suggestions:

1. Plan ahead. Read labels. Write out menus. See Appendix B for menus to help you through the Common Foods Elimination Diet.

Don't start the diet the week before Christmas or another holiday. Don't start it when you're traveling or visiting friends or relatives.

2. When you begin reintroducing foods, give your child a small portion of the eliminated food for breakfast. If no reaction occurs, let your child eat more of the food for a morning snack, lunch, afternoon snack, supper, and bedtime snack.

3. Continue following the rest of the Common Foods Elimination Diet while testing the individual foods.

4. If your child shows an obvious reaction after eating a food, don't give him any more of that food. Wait until the reaction subsides (usually twenty-four to forty-eight hours) before you add another food.

5. If a food really bothers your child, you can shorten his reaction by giving him two tablets of aspirin-free Alka-Seltzer Gold (in the gold foil package) in a glass of water. The alkalizing effect is thought to change the body's acidity level slightly, which can improve symptoms—sometimes dramatically. If this settles your child down, you can use it occasionally when your child is off his diet and feeling awful and driving you nuts.

6. If you find that a food causes your child's symptoms, keep it out of his diet for three to four weeks, then cautiously try it again. If he still reacts to the food, avoid it again for several months. Many food-sensitive people find that they can eat a small amount of the food every four to seven days.

If your head is spinning and you're thinking there's no way to sell your family and child on eating this diet, you could try limiting the elimination diet to just milk, artificial colors, chocolate, and sugar. Then you could test the other foods at a later date. But the ideal way is to carry out the Common Foods Elimination Diet. Pediatric allergist and ADD/ADHD expert Doris Rapp, M.D., once made the statement that if you have five nails in the bottom of your boot, removing just two of them doesn't improve the pain very much. It's the same with the elimination diet. If your child is sensitive to five foods, removing two from his diet might not significantly improve his symptoms.

THE CAVEMAN DIET

The Caveman Diet avoids all the foods your child normally eats at least once a week, whether you think they may be a culprit or not. Most children do not need the Caveman Diet. However, if you tried the Common Foods Elimination Diet and your child improved when the foods were withheld and reacted to most of the foods tested, but still has significant symptoms even without those foods in his diet, you'll want to search for more food culprits. Since your child is most likely to be allergic to foods he eats most often, custom-design a diet that avoids all foods he eats at least once a week.

For example, four-year-old Paul was extremely hyperactive and also had autistic tendencies. He was not close to being potty-trained. His nose was constantly stuffy. His temper tantrums were frequent and severe. His parents had tried the Common Foods Elimination Diet and learned that milk caused itchiness and tantrums, artificial colors caused excessive chatter and weeping, corn caused excessive chatter and bloating, and orange juice caused Paul to become antsy and uncooperative. Paul was better after avoiding these foods, but his problems were so severe that Paul's parents decided to try the Caveman Diet to see if they could identify other food culprits. Sure enough, Paul was sensitive to strawberries, bananas, apples, and beef. Here's how Paul's parents set up the Caveman Diet. They made a list of all the foods that Paul ate less than once a week. Then they built a diet and menus around these foods. Here are the foods Paul could eat on his Caveman Diet (your child's list will be unique for him):

> Fruits: Watermelon, cantaloupe, honeydew melon, pears, blueberries, raspberries, cherries, grapes, pineapple, mangos, apricots
>
> Vegetables: Sweet potatoes, carrots, squash, broccoli, asparagus, cabbage, celery
>
> Meats: Turkey; fresh fish and seafood—tuna, salmon, shrimp, crabs, etc.; lamb; venison; rabbit; duck; goose

Grains: Amaranth, quinoa, buckwheat, potato starch; avoid all
  grains including wheat, rye, barley, oats, and rice
Unprocessed nuts and seeds: Walnuts, pecans, cashews, almonds,
  pistachios, sunflower seeds
Nut butters: Cashew butter, almond butter
Vegetable oils: Canola, sunflower, or safflower oils
Beverages: Bottled or spring water

PLAYING THE DIET GAME WITH YOUR CHILD

It's not easy to follow the Common Foods Elimination Diet or the Caveman Diet, but the benefits may be so spectacular that it's worth all the time and effort. Your child will need a lot of help to stay on his diet. He is likely to say, "No way! I won't do this dumb diet. I'd have to give up all my favorite foods. I can't live without hot dogs, ice cream, orange juice, and peanut butter. I won't do it!"

Here's how to get your child to stay on his diet. First, show him on the calendar how long the diet will last. You can say, "It's not forever—just a couple of weeks. I know you can do that."

Second, explain to him how much better he will feel and act. You can say, "I know you hate it when your nose is all stuffed up and your legs ache. And I also know how hard you try at school and how much you would like to get better grades. This diet may help you feel, act, and learn better." Third, enlist his help in planning his diet. You could say, "Here are the foods you can eat. I need your help in planning the menus. I'll also need your help in preparing snacks and meals."

Fourth, set up a system of rewards. Say to your child, "You like playing games and earning prizes. Would you like to earn a prize every day if you eat only the foods allowed on your diet? And at the end of the diet you can earn a big prize. Let's talk about what prizes you'd like to earn."

Keep track of the foods he eats at each meal. Every time he eats the allowed foods, he can earn a star. Then at the end of each day, if he has earned at least six stars, he earns a small prize. At the end of two weeks, if he hasn't cheated on his diet, he can earn a big prize. You will deserve a prize, too! After the diet is completed, treat yourself to new clothes, a movie, lunch with friends—something you'll look forward to. Of course, the biggest reward of all would be a marked improvement in your child's behavior!

WAY 4.
ADD ESSENTIAL
FATTY ACIDS TO
YOUR CHILD'S DIET

So much has been said in recent years about eliminating fat from one's diet that it has become ingrained in America's consciousness that fats are the enemy. Because of this, most of us do our best to eliminate foods high in fat, even plant foods naturally high in fat, from our families' diets. The problem is that some fats are actually good for you and particularly for your child. Essential fatty acids are necessary for your child's optimal health. Deficiency of these fatty acids has been found to be a factor in some children with ADD and ADHD.

Does your child show symptoms of marginal essential fatty acid depletion? Answer yes or no to the following questions about your child's symptoms:

1. Is your child excessively thirsty?
2. Does your child urinate frequently?
3. Does your child have dry, flaking skin?

4. Does your child have dry, strawlike, or unmanageable hair?
5. Does your child have dandruff?
6. Does your child have brittle, soft, or splitting fingernails?
7. Does your child have small, hard bumps on the backs of his arms, elbows, or thighs?

If you answered yes to more than one of these questions, your child may have a marginal essential fatty acid deficiency. This chapter will explain what essential fatty acids are, how they affect your child's ADD/ADHD, and how you can supplement your child's diet with them.

WHAT ARE ESSENTIAL FATTY ACIDS?

Our bodies are composed of billions of cells—units of life—of various shapes and functions. Each cell is surrounded by a waterproof membrane composed of special types of fats that separate the watery contents of the cell from the watery fluid outside the cell. These special fats are called *essential fatty acids (EFAs)*. They are vital nutrients that come directly and *only from our foods*. Humans and other mammals cannot manufacture these fatty acids.

There are two families of EFAs, the omega-3s and the omega-6s. The two families are not interchangeable. Your body can't make omega-3 fatty acids from omega-6 fatty acids or vice versa. The omega-6 family starts with linoleic acid (LA), while the omega-3 family starts with alpha-linolenic acid (ALA). LA and ALA are both made up of eighteen carbon atoms strung together rather like beads in a necklace. While most of the "beads" are linked by a single link, LA has two double links (double bonds) while ALA has three double links. The position of the first double bond is the sixth carbon atom for LA and the third carbon atom for ALA—hence the terms omega-3 and omega-6. LA and ALA then undergo several transformations in which they are lengthened twice by two carbons and more double bonds inserted. The double bonds are important because they cause kinks in the fatty acids molecule. While saturated fatty acids have no kinks and thus pack closely together in the membrane, the kinks in the essential fatty acids prevent the molecules from becoming packed together and allow the membrane to be fluid. Other members of the omega-3 family include eicosapentaenoic acid (EPA) and docosahexaenoic acid (DHA). In addition to linoleic acid, the omega-6 family of fatty acids includes cis-linoleic acid, gamma-linolenic acid (GLA), dihomogammalinolenic acid (DGLA), and arachidonic acid (AA).

Essential fatty acids are crucial for two reasons. First, the balance between the omega-3 fatty acids and the omega-6 fatty acids affects the properties of the cell membrane and the ability of molecules to enter and exit the cell or to bind to receptors in the membrane. Your child's body also uses longer-chain omega-3 and omega-6 fatty acids to manufacture different series of hormonelike chemicals, including prostaglandins. Prostaglandins (PGs) help cells communicate with one another. Long-chain omega-6 fatty acids (AA) and especially long chain omega-3 fatty acids (DHA) are more concentrated in the brain and retina than in other cells. They play vital roles in brain and nerve function. They're also critical for proper functioning of the immune system. In fact, a study of children with recurrent respiratory infections reported that those children who received a supplement of LA and ALA had fewer infections.[1] If your child is low in these critical fatty acids, the odds of the game of life are unfairly stacked against him: He is starting out the game without a full deck of cards!

ESSENTIAL FATTY ACIDS AND ADHD

In 1986 scientists reported that boys with ADHD had lower levels of critical EFAs in their blood than a group of children exhibiting "normal" behavior.[2] These children also reported excessive thirst and frequent urination—two important symptoms of EFA deficiency. They also had more allergies, visual problems, ear infections, colds, and learning problems than did children with normal behavior. Scientists have known for many years that a deficiency of omega-6 fatty acids leads to impaired growth, dry, scaly skin, excessive thirst, and frequent urination in animals. More recently, researchers also studied monkeys, rats, and mice who were fed a very low omega-3 diet as fetuses and during lactation and adulthood.[3] The animals had lower levels of omega-3 EFAs in the blood and brain. The animals showed excessive thirst, frequent urination, visual disturbances, decreased learning abilities, and abnormal behavior.

In the early 1990s, researchers studied children with ADHD and their fatty acid status. About 40 percent of the boys with ADHD reported many symptoms of EFA deficiency. Boys with many symptoms had lower blood plasma levels of critical omega-3 (DHA) and omega-6 (AA) fatty acids than controls with normal behavior. However, children with ADHD but without symptoms had plasma levels comparable to the boys without ADHD. The same is thought to be true for children with ADD, but this has not yet been studied. The reason for the lower EFA levels is not known. Ongoing research is studying whether or not supplements of EFAs will increase EFA blood levels, improve deficiency symptoms, and improve behavior.

ADDING EFAS TO YOUR CHILD'S DIET

If your child has symptoms of EFA deficiency, here are some easy, inexpensive ways to add essential fatty acids—especially omega-3s—to your family's diet. This may benefit all family members, because omega-3 fatty acids, especially those in fish oils, reduce the risk of cardiovascular disease, asthma, arthritis, high blood pressure, and autoimmune disorders.

Use pure, cold-pressed soy (unless your child is sensitive to soy) or canola oils (1 to 2 tablespoons each day). These are excellent sources of ALA. Use the oils to make homemade salad dressings. Stir these oils into spaghetti sauce, chili, etc. Use them to make pasta salad. Baking with them is fine. But avoid using them for frying because the fragile molecules are damaged by the high heat and oxygen. To protect the fragile molecules after opening a new bottle of oil, squeeze the contents of a 50 international units (IU) capsule of vitamin E (natural alpha-tocopherol, not alpha-tocopherol acetate) into the oil and slowly disperse it. Don't shake the bottle because you don't want to mix air bubbles with the oil. Then keep the bottle refrigerated.

An even richer source of ALA, the parent of the omega-3 family, is flaxseed oil. You can give your child 1 to 3 teaspoons of flaxseed oil every day. Keep the flaxseed oil refrigerated and add the contents of a capsule of vitamin E as described above. Use within a couple of months because you want the oil to be as fresh as possible. Or you can buy the seeds themselves. Grind a tablespoon of the flaxseed in a small coffee or spice mill. Sprinkle over cereal and salads or stir into applesauce. The seeds are an excellent source of omega-3 fatty acids, magnesium, and fiber.

Beans are another good source of omega-3 essential fatty acids (ALA)—especially soy, navy, kidney, pinto, and red beans. So is tofu if your child is not sensitive to soy. Cold-water fish such as salmon, fresh tuna, mackerel, or sardines are excellent sources of long-chain omega-3 fatty acids (EPA and DHA), although some children might turn up their noses at them. Unfortunately, fish sticks and sole are not good sources of omega-3 fatty acids; not to mention that they are usually prepared with hydrogenated and partially hydrogenated fats.

Decreasing saturated fats in your child's diet is also important because they interfere with essential fatty acid metabolism. Like most Americans, you may be consuming too much saturated fat found in fatty meats, butter, whole milk, lard, and coconut oil. It's hard to cut down on these fats unless you start baking, steaming, roasting, and broiling your foods and begin eating more fish and chicken and less bacon, hamburger, and pork products.

In addition to saturated fats your child is probably also consuming hydrogenated or partially hydrogenated vegetable oils. These fats don't have kinks in their molecules, so these straight fatty acids pack next to each other, making cell membranes less fluid and stiffer. This type of fat is found in many commercially prepared foods, including margarine, cream soup, Triscuits, Wheat Thins, saltines, and hundreds of other foods you find on your supermarket shelf. So read all labels and decrease those foods that contain hydrogenated or partially hydrogenated oils.

Compare the following dinner menus. The first three meals are low in EFAs. The second three are healthy alternatives high in EFAs.

Dinner Menus Low in EFAs

Dinner #1
Broiled steak
Iceberg lettuce with fat-free dressing
French fries
Green beans
Ice cream

Dinner #2
Spaghetti
Jell-O with fruit
Garlic bread (white)
Apple pie

Dinner #3
Chili (no beans)
Saltines
Ice cream and cookies

Dinner Menus High in EFAs

Dinner #1
Broiled salmon*
Green leafy salad* with salad dressing made from soy* or canola oil*
Baked potato
Watermelon

Dinner #2
Waldorf salad made with walnuts*
Spaghetti with added soy* or canola oils*
Whole-wheat bread with all-fruit jam
Sliced fresh peaches

---

*An excellent source of omega-3 fatty acids.

Dinner #3
Chili (with kidney beans* and extra soy* or canola oil*)
Whole-wheat crackers
Fresh fruit cup
Apple pie (see recipe in Part 3)

SIGNS OF EFA DEFICIENCY

At present, blood tests for EFA depletion are available only through special research labs and only a few commercial labs. They're expensive—$300 to $400. Even if you had the tests performed, your doctor probably would not know how to interpret the scores. Many doctors who recommend EFAs to their patients don't depend on lab tests. Instead, they ask patients about symptoms and look for physical signs of a marginal deficiency, followed by a trial of EFA supplementation. Symptoms of an essential fatty acid deficiency include excessive thirst; frequent urination; dry skin; dry, unmanageable hair; dandruff; brittle nails; and small, hard bumps on the backs of the arms or thighs.

I get many e-mail messages from parents about the fabulous results they have gotten from supplementing their children's diets with fatty acids. One mother reported her son's excessive thirst and exhausting behavior:

John's always been thirsty. As a preschooler, John would sneak into the kitchen and drink glass after glass of milk and orange juice. We had to stop buying orange juice because he would spirit off the container and could go through the better part of a gallon.

John screamed from birth, crying wildly if he was not carried around in an upright position, until he could scoot at about nine months. At ten months he was walking. At fifteen months he started to pound his head when he became enraged. Anything could set him off and did. (Mom turned left instead of right; Dad went into the next room; someone picked up one of

---

*An excellent source of omega-3 fatty acids.

fifteen toys he had around him.) No form of behavioral management was
helpful.

Last summer a psychiatrist medicated him. Then he became lethargic.
We've lost a lot of the joy and social ability with these medications. The
medications have also blunted his intelligence and ability to learn. They also
seemed to impair his memory.

John's been on flaxseed oil now for two weeks. His thirst has really
improved. He also seems calmer and more focused.

The above is representative of the several stories I am told day after day
about the effects of EFA supplementation. Following is yet another example. Barb relates her experiences with her eleven-year-old daughter,
Sarah:

Sarah is a sweet, loving, and intelligent child with severe ADHD symptoms.
She has been on a changing regimen of medicines since first grade. Despite
wonderful, caring teachers and lots of help at home, Sarah is failing all her
classes. Her self-esteem has dwindled to nothing.

Sarah has just about all of the symptoms of essential fatty acid deficiencies:
excessive thirst, frequent urination, dry skin, dry hair, dandruff, brittle
nails, and small, white bumps on the backs of her arms. Her psychiatrist
thought she might have lupus because of some of her skin conditions. I took
her to an endocrinologist and all the tests were negative. She was also checked
for diabetes because of her excessive thirst and frequent urination.

We've added soy oil to her diet plus 3 teaspoons of flaxseed oil. The change
has been dramatic. Her thirst diminished within two days and her skin and
hair are much better. Her behavior is much improved, too. Her teacher is
amazed at the changes in Sarah.

Many parents report stories like Sarah's—they've had their children
tested for diabetes because of the child's excessive thirst and frequent urination. If your child has these symptoms, discuss them thoroughly with
your doctor. He may want to test your child for diabetes. The results will
probably be normal.

Essential fatty acids seem to be one important piece of ADHD and ADD children's jigsaw puzzles. If you walk down the aisle in your drugstore or grocery you may be surprised at how many different products there are for dry skin, dry hair, and dandruff. Hair and skin should both be lustrous without the use of creams and lotions. Some adults take their beverage of choice everywhere they go because they're constantly thirsty. EFA deficiency may be much more common in Americans than researchers once thought.

Your child may benefit from increasing EFAs in his diet. If you want your child to look sharp, feel sharp, act sharp, and enjoy good health, make sure he gets adequate amounts of essential fatty acids, especially omega-3 oils. Your whole family may benefit.

WAY 5.
CHOOSE VITAMINS,
MINERALS, AND OTHER
SUPPLEMENTS CAREFULLY

Parents often ask, "Is there a vitamin, mineral, or other supplement I can give my child to replace Ritalin?" Unfortunately, it's usually not that simple, but certain supplements may help.

Answer yes or no to the following questions pertaining to your child's need for supplementation.

1. Is your child a picky eater?
2. Does your child eat fewer than two to four servings of fruits and three to five servings of vegetables a day?
3. Does your child consume mostly white flour and no whole grains?
4. Is your child a "sugarholic"?
5. Does your child eat essentially the same few foods every day?
6. Does your child drink more than three 8-ounce glasses of milk every day, leaving little room for complete meals?

7. Does he drink more than 12 ounces of fruit juice every day, leaving little room for complete meals?

The use of vitamins and minerals to alleviate various physical and mental symptoms has been controversial. Most of the medical establishment used to declare that anyone who eats a good, balanced diet needs no additional vitamins or minerals. If you asked your doctor whether you should take a daily multivitamin preparation, she may have answered that although the only thing it will hurt is your pocketbook, it won't make you healthier. And if you asked whether larger doses might be helpful for depression or allergies, your doctor probably thought you were "one of those health-food nuts" and gave you a lecture on the harmful effects of too many vitamins.

Although there has been a lot of discussion in the popular press and on the Internet about the pros and cons of vitamin, mineral, and other supplements for children with ADD or ADHD, there haven't been many scientific studies of the effects of these nutrients on ADD and ADHD. For example, the use of a multivitamin/mineral supplement containing RDA amounts hasn't been studied in children with ADD/ADHD. However, there have been scientific reports of the positive effects of a multivitamin/ mineral supplement on intelligence and conduct.[1] It is hoped that scientists will study this soon in children with ADD/ADHD. In the meantime, parents can try a multivitamin/mineral supplement free of artificial color and flavor, and containing RDA amounts. It should be kept in mind, though, that B vitamins may worsen symptoms in some children. This will be discussed later in the chapter.

On the other side of the debate is a group of doctors who claim they have found a whole new approach to treating psychiatric and medical problems through using moderate to large doses of nutrients to compensate for biochemical imbalances. In the middle was the patient, not knowing what to believe but anxious to get better. Times are changing because patients have demanded more information and advice from their doctors. More than eighty-five medical schools offer classes in alternative therapies.

What is a vitamin, and why is there all this controversy? A vitamin is an organic (carbon-containing) substance found in plants and animals in varying quantities. Each vitamin is absolutely necessary for proper growth and maintenance of health. Except for a few vitamins (which, technically, are not true vitamins), your child's body cannot make these chemicals itself. Your child must obtain them from his diet or in vitamin supplements.

Six basic nutrients are essential for life: carbohydrates, fats, proteins, vitamins, minerals, and water. If you think of your child's body as a car engine, carbohydrates, fats, and proteins are the gasoline giving you energy. But vitamins are the spark plugs, oil, and grease; without them, your child's body can't function. They are catalysts for all the biochemical reactions in your child's body.

There are two kinds of vitamins: fat-soluble and water-soluble. Fat-soluble vitamins A, D, E, and K dissolve only in fat and are therefore stored in the body. Taken in excess, they can be harmful. Water-soluble B vitamins and vitamin C dissolve in water so that excess amounts not needed by the body are excreted in the urine. But these vitamins must be obtained daily.

Vitamins were isolated and identified during the first half of the twentieth century. Considerable interest and enthusiasm were aroused by their ability to cure deficiency diseases such as scurvy and beriberi. When antibiotics began to crowd the scene in the 1940s, catching all the attention, the excitement surrounding vitamins diminished. To safeguard our health, the Food and Nutrition Board of the National Academy of Sciences was established in 1941. It came up with a list of minimum daily nutrient requirements, which has been revised over the years and is now referred to as the Recommended Dietary Allowance (RDA). These requirements, however, are adequate only to prevent deficiency; they do not appear to be the levels required by the body for its function at optimal levels.

Nutrition-oriented doctors agree with the medical establishment that following the RDA will generally prevent vitamin-deficiency diseases. But they believe there is an optimal dosage of each nutrient for each person that allows a person to function physically and mentally at his or her best. In their opinion, an average value (such as the RDA) doesn't consider that each person is biochemically unique. They contend that a variety of factors determine how much of a given nutrient a person needs, including height and weight, age, activity level, stress, infection, and such environmental conditions as air pollution.

What especially concerns these doctors is that not only do many American children and adults not eat a good diet (see Way 1), but they really don't know what a good diet is. And the average doctor will not know much more than his patients. Nutrition-oriented doctors are also concerned that modern processing of whole foods robs the consumer of essential nutrients, even though manufacturers attempt to undo the damage by enriching their products with a few essential vitamins and minerals.

Perhaps the most hotly debated issue is the use of megavitamins—large doses (more than ten times the RDA) to prevent and treat physical and mental problems; for example, whether or not large doses of vitamin C will help prevent colds or ease their severity.

Traditional and nutrition-oriented doctors are concerned about self-treatment by people who don't really know what they're doing, especially as large doses of fat-soluble vitamins can cause problems. They're worried that some patients will figure if they take their vitamins, it doesn't matter what they eat or do. So if your child is a picky eater, giving him a multivitamin that contains RDA amounts for various nutrients may help, but *the goal always should be to take steps to improve the diet*. Way 1 will give you lots of ideas.

Where does this leave you, the frustrated parent? If you can, find an experienced nutritionally oriented doctor to help you. This doctor can save you lots of time and money in the long run by closely monitoring symptoms, diet, and hair, blood, and urine levels of various nutrients. Don't blindly supplement your child with large doses of vitamins and minerals over a long period of time. Nutrients interact with each other and with prescription medication. It's wrong to think, "If one pill makes my child feel better, ten pills will help even more." You can make your child worse.

If someone recommends that you take so much of such and such vitamin, be sure the information is reliable. I've been appalled at some of the practices I've seen in one health-food store. Once a salesperson offered my children chewable vitamin pills as though they were candy: "Here, kids you'll love the taste, and it's good for you." Another time a salesperson was pushing chewable vitamin C tablets at the checkout counter. She told the woman ahead of me to try one of the samples. When the woman remarked how tasty it was, the salesperson sold her a large bottle with the advice,

"Eat them all day, they can't possibly harm you, and they'll give you so much energy." What she neglected to mention to the unsuspecting customer is that too much vitamin C causes gas and diarrhea!

Another concern about vitamin and mineral supplements are the fillers, binders, dyes, and flavorings. You'll have to read the labels carefully. It's common for supplements for kids to contain artificial color and flavors, corn, and/or sugar. One frustrated mother wrote: "My son is very sensitive to artificial colors. When I started to read all labels more carefully, I was amazed that his multivitamin tablet was artificially colored and flavored."

Minerals are inorganic chemicals—they don't contain the element carbon. Some, like calcium and magnesium, are needed by your body in fairly large amounts, others are needed in small but critical amounts. Still other minerals, like lead and aluminum (see Way 9), can be very toxic inside your child's body.

As with vitamins, deficiencies of certain minerals can cause mild to severe symptoms. Too much of a good mineral can be devastating, too. Can laboratory tests tell your doctor if your child is getting too much or too little of specific vitamins and minerals? The answer is yes for some nutrients and no for others. Blood tests are available for the status of many vitamins. A hair analysis can give your doctor some important information about toxic elements such as lead, cadmium, mercury, and aluminum. All that is needed is 1 to 2 tablespoons of hair clippings from the nape of your child's neck, clipped close to the scalp. Measuring zinc in plasma and red blood cells may be helpful. Magnesium can also be assessed in red blood cells. Measuring plasma calcium is not very helpful, because when calcium levels fall low, the body takes calcium from the bones to keep the level of calcium in the bloodstream in balance; so though plasma levels may be normal, the body may still be deficient.

SCIENTIFIC STUDIES

As you read about more vitamin and mineral supplements in this book and other resources, how can you decide which supplements have been well studied and are worth trying and which ones are not? The investigation of a drug or nutrient often begins with an open study. In an open study, both the researchers and the patients know that they're getting the "real" thing. For children with ADHD the behavior scores usually improve because the parents, teachers, and children are expecting a positive result. This is called the placebo effect. If a drug or nutrient has been found to be beneficial in an open trial, the next step is to conduct a double-blind, placebo-controlled test. In this kind of study half the group is given a placebo (a dummy, lookalike pill) and the other half the real medicine or nutrient. Parents do not know whether their children are taking the active or placebo supplement. Further, researchers in contact with the parents are also "blind" as to which child is in which group. These kinds of studies should be conducted by independent research groups at medical centers or universities. Careful statistical analysis of the results is crucial. These results should be published in well-respected journals. Supplements for children with ADHD could be studied inexpensively, and these studies would give us all better information. Keeping all that in mind, here is information about vitamin, mineral, and other supplements.

VITAMIN SUPPLEMENTS

Here is some basic information about several vitamins that will help you decide whether your child should try the supplements.

B Vitamins

B vitamins include several water-soluble compounds that are grouped together by scientists because they work together in your child's body. The amounts needed are small. The table on page 99 shows the RDAs for some of the B-complex vitamins for children.

Good sources of B vitamins include liver; whole-grain flours, cereals, and breads; enriched flour (vitamin B_6 is not added back to enriched flour) and cereals; peas; beans; and green leafy vegetables. B-complex vitamins are easily destroyed—some by heat and light, some by food processing. You could try a B-complex supplement that provides about 25 milligrams

RDAs for B-Complex Vitamins

B VITAMIN	AGE RANGE (YEARS)	RDA
Thiamin (B$_1$)	1 to 3	.5 milligram
	4 to 8	.6 milligram
	9 to 13	.9 milligram
	14 and over	1.2 milligrams (boys)
		1.0 milligram (girls)
Riboflavin (B$_2$)	1 to 3	.5 milligram
	4 to 8	.6 milligram
	9 to 13	.9 milligram
	14 and over	1.2 milligrams (boys)
		1.0 milligram (girls)
Niacin	1 to 3	6 milligrams
	4 to 8	8 milligrams
	9 to 13	12 milligrams
	14 and over	16 milligrams (boys)
		14 milligrams (girls)
Pyridoxine (B$_6$)	1 to 3	.5 milligram
	4 to 8	.6 milligram
	9 to 13	1.0 milligram
	14 and over	1.3 milligrams (boys)
		1.2 milligrams (girls)
Folic acid	1 to 3	150 micrograms
	4 to 8	200 micrograms
	9 to 13	300 micrograms
	14 and over	400 micrograms
Vitamin B$_{12}$	1 to 3	.9 microgram
	4 to 8	1.2 micrograms
	9 to 13	1.8 micrograms
	14 and over	2.4 micrograms

of thiamin, niacin, and B$_6$ plus all the other B vitamins. But some hyperactive children are *worse* on large or megadoses of vitamins, especially B vitamins. Expert Leo Galland, M.D., has written:

> *The B-vitamins are especially tricky. Some children are allergic to the yeast used in making most B-complex tablets or capsules. Others simply have adverse reactions to the B-vitamins themselves. I've found that hyperactive children are generally also hypersensitive: they overreact to stimuli, whether chemical, sensory, or emotional.*[2]

Arnold Brenner, M.D., carried out an interesting study of selected B-complex vitamins in hyperactive children.[3] He gave 100 hyperactive children three-day trials of large doses of thiamin (B$_1$), calcium pantothenate (pantothenic acid—vitamin B$_5$), pyridoxine (B$_6$), or placebo. The three-day trials were followed by double-blind, placebo-controlled studies. Eight children dramatically responded to thiamin (100 mg taken four times a day). Nine children responded to 300 milligrams of vitamin B$_6$. Another four children needed larger doses of vitamin B$_6$ before they responded. But half the children who responded to vitamin B$_1$ worsened when given vitamin B$_6$. Conversely, half the children who responded positively to vitamin B$_6$ worsened when given vitamin B$_1$. So it is tricky. If possible find a professional who has had experience in working with children with ADHD. If you decide to try B vitamins on your own, try them cautiously one at a time and stop any B vitamins that worsen any symptoms.

Vitamin C

Vitamin C is important for the formation of blood vessels, red blood cells, bones, teeth, and connective tissue. It is also believed to fight viral infections and to reduce the effects on the body of allergy-causing substances.

The RDA for vitamin C is 40 milligrams in children four to six, 45 milligrams in children ages seven to ten, 50 milligrams for those between the ages of eleven and fourteen, and 60 milligrams for those fifteen and over. Citrus fruits are especially high in vitamin C, but other fruits and vegetables also have high quantities. Because vitamin C is easily destroyed by heat, sunlight, air, drying, and long storage, you should, if possible, buy your vitamin-C-containing produce fresh and eat the foods raw. Bioflavonoids, water-soluble compounds found in several fruits and vegetables, including those containing vitamin C, are essential for the proper use of vitamin C. They are much more concentrated in the whole edible part of the fruit than in the juice. The table below lists some good natural sources of vitamin C.

If your child has allergies or frequent, severe colds, vitamin C may help his resistance. Studies have shown that children who take larger doses than the RDA for vitamin C have less severe colds.[4] The dose for children is 500 mg once or twice each day. Most vitamin C supplements are made from corn. They are available in liquids (beware of sugar, colorings, and flavorings), chewable tablets (same problems), tablets, and powder. The powder is the cheapest and can be stirred into juices. Nausea, gas, and diarrhea are signs that your child is taking too much. Reduce the dose.

Some Good Natural Sources of Vitamin C

Orange (1 medium)	90 milligrams
Broccoli (½ cup)	8 milligrams
Orange juice (½ cup)	60 milligrams
Strawberries (¾ cup)	66 milligrams
Cantaloupe (½ medium)	66 milligrams
Brussels sprouts (½ cup, cooked)	57 milligrams
Grapefruit (½ medium)	53 milligrams
Tangerine (1 medium)	35 milligrams
Cauliflower (½ cup, steamed)	33 milligrams
Beef liver (4 ounces)	31 milligrams
Cabbage (½ cup, shredded raw)	22 milligrams

MINERALS

Supplementing with minerals in those with ADHD is another strategy that needs many more careful studies. In Poland, researchers studied magnesium, zinc, copper, iron, and calcium levels in plasma, red blood cells, urine, and hair in fifty hyperactive children ages four to thirteen.[5] The average concentration of all these minerals was lower compared with a group of healthy children with no behavior problems.

Calcium

Calcium is the most abundant mineral in the body. It is located primarily in the bones and teeth. In addition to its role in growth, it is essential for nervous-system functioning, a normal heart rhythm, and blood clotting. The RDA for children ages one to ten is 800 milligrams a day. It is 1,200 milligrams daily for older children. The table on page 103 lists some good food sources of calcium.

If your child dislikes milk and cheese products or is sensitive to dairy products, then it's imperative that he take calcium supplements to build strong teeth and bones. Calcium may also have a calming effect on his behavior and promote sleep at night. The dosage is 500 to 1,000 milligrams of calcium carbonate, depending on the age of the child, in liquid or chewable tablets. (Avoid supplements of dolomite or bone meal, which may contain low levels of lead. Avoid Tums, which contain talc and sugar.) Too much calcium affects the absorption of other minerals.

Magnesium

If your hyperactive, irritable child has trouble getting to sleep, experiences muscle twitches or muscle cramps, has poor concentration, experiences frequent constipation, and/or wets the bed, magnesium supplements may help. Magnesium is an important mineral that serves as a cofactor in many chemical reactions in the body. When magnesium is deficient, children may have neurological and psychiatric problems. The RDA for magnesium is 120 milligrams for children between the ages of four and six, 170 milligrams for children ages seven to ten, 270 milligrams for boys between the ages of eleven and fourteen, and 280 milligrams for girls between the

Some Good Food Sources of Calcium	
Milk (1 cup)	288 milligrams
Yogurt (1 cup)	174 milligrams
Tofu (½ cup)	128 milligrams
Spinach (½ cup cooked)	83 milligrams
Cottage cheese (½ cup)	70 milligrams
Broccoli, raw (½ cup)	55 milligrams

ages of eleven and fourteen. Refining foods greatly reduces the magnesium content. Good food sources include whole grains, nuts, seafood, fresh vegetables, and fruit.

Magnesium supplements may have a positive effect on your child's allergies and his behavior. Magnesium calms many hyperactive children and helps with their sleep. Two new studies suggest that magnesium deficiency is common in children with ADHD (94 percent showed low levels of magnesium in hair, red blood cells, and/or blood serum). In a second study, the researchers supplemented fifty children with ADHD and magnesium deficiency with magnesium (200 milligrams per day), which led to a significant decrease in hyperactivity.[6] More double-blind, placebo-controlled studies need to be conducted.

You can look for one sign of a magnesium deficiency in your child. It's called Cvostek's sign. Just tap lightly in the hollow of your child's cheek, halfway between the corner of his mouth and the bottom of his ear. If the upper lip beneath his nose twitches or jumps, the test is considered "positive" and usually indicates a magnesium deficiency. It's impossible to fake this test.[7] Children with chronic allergic problems and yeast problems often have a positive Cvostek's sign and improve on magnesium supplements.

Magnesium chloride and magnesium citrate are two well-absorbed supplement forms. The dosage should be about 200 to 600 milligrams of magnesium per day. Multiply your child's weight by six, and that's the amount of supplemental magnesium, in milligrams, to try.[8] For example, a fifty-pound child would need 300 milligrams of magnesium a day. Side effects of taking high dosages of magnesium include diarrhea, indicating the dose should be reduced. Supplementing magnesium is a safe, cheap, easy kind of therapy to try. Children with kidney problems should take magnesium only under their doctor's close supervision.

Zinc

Zinc is another vital mineral that is a cofactor in many key metabolic pathways. A recent study compared blood serum zinc levels of children with ADHD and children without. Blood serum zinc levels of the children with ADHD were significantly lower than the levels in the children without ADHD.[9] The RDA for zinc in children between the ages of four and ten is 10 milligrams. For boys between the ages of eleven and fourteen, the RDA is 15 milligrams, and for girls in that age range it is 12 milligrams. If your child has a loss of appetite, slow growth, slow wound healing, altered taste perception, and/or white spots on his fingernails, he may have a marginal zinc deficiency. Good food sources include eggs, liver, shellfish, wheat germ, beef, dark-meat turkey, nuts, and seeds. Taking 10 milligrams of zinc as part of a multimineral preparation for two months may improve his health and behavior. Taking too much zinc is harmful because it decreases the absorption of other vital minerals. According to Leo Galland, M.D., the multimineral tablet containing 10 milligrams of zinc should include 1 milligram of copper, 10 milligrams of manganese, 75 milligrams of selenium, 200 micrograms of chromium, and 200 micrograms of molybdenum.[10]

If your child has a sore throat and a developing cold, you may reduce the duration and symptoms of the cold by giving your child zinc lozenges to suck every few hours. Studies have shown that adults who use Cold-Eeze, a new commercial zinc lozenge, have less severe colds that last for fewer days.[11] However, a recent study in children has not shown the same results.[12] More studies are needed. Unfortunately, Cold-Eeze also contains corn syrup, sugar, and citrus flavoring. Your health-food store will have zinc lozenges that don't contain sugar.

Selenium

Selenium is a trace mineral that plays an important role in many metabolic processes, including strengthening the immune system. Although we need oxygen to exist, some forms of oxygen molecules generate "free radicals," which can damage tissues. Antioxidants are compounds that protect the body from the effects of free radicals. Selenium is one of many antioxidants. It's a trace mineral that is greatly reduced by refining foods. Good food sources include seafood, liver, and meat. Grains are good sources only if they are grown on selenium-rich fields. If your child has many chemical sensitivities, selenium may help. Look for a multimineral supplement that contains 75 micrograms of selenium. Do not exceed this amount, as selenium is toxic in large amounts.

OTHER SUPPLEMENTS

There are supplements in addition to vitamins and minerals that may be helpful in the treatment of ADD or ADHD. Again, not many of them have been formally studied for their effects on children with these disorders. We are in desperate need of studies of these supplements so that parents can make informed choices. Currently, supplements are apparently safe and nontoxic in the recommended doses.

Lactobacillus Acidophilus, Bifidus, and Plantarum

If your child has taken multiple prescriptions of antibiotics, taking supplements of "good" bacteria may help restore the balance between bacteria and yeast in the intestines. (See Way 6.) Most supplements should be kept refrigerated. Choose powders or capsules but not pills. Follow the directions on the bottle.

Glyconutritional Supplements

Several kinds of special sugar molecules help cells communicate with one another. In two open studies of these glyconutrients, children with ADHD were given these supplements.[13] Their inattention and hyperactivity-impulsivity scores improved. This is another area that needs to be investigated with double-blind, placebo-controlled studies.

Chinese Herbs

Here's some interesting information about Chinese herbs and ADHD. In an open study, Chinese scientists compared use of a Chinese herbal preparation* to Ritalin in hyperactive children for one to three months.[14] The clinical symptoms disappeared in twenty-three of eighty children taking the herbal medicine. Six of twenty children taking Ritalin improved completely. Forty-six children improved on the herbs. The rate of effectiveness was 86 percent for the group taking the herbs while the effective rate was 90 percent for the group taking Ritalin. Interestingly, the children receiving the herbs improved their IQ and also had less bed-wetting. In addition, there were fewer side effects for the children taking the Chinese herbs than for those taking Ritalin. Obviously this possible treatment needs to be followed up with careful double-blind, placebo-controlled studies.

In another Chinese open study, scientists gave 100 hyperactive children Tiaoshen liquor that consisted of Chinese herbal drugs.[15] Behavior improved greatly, inattention improved, and their academic grades went up. The effective rate was 94 percent. Again, this study needs to be confirmed by double-blind, placebo-controlled studies.

Other Supplements

Other popular supplements have been suggested as a replacement for Ritalin to help children with ADHD, including blue-green algae, St.-John's-wort, Pycnogenol, grape-seed extract, DMAE (dimethylaminoethanol bitartrate), colloidal minerals, and echinacea. There are anecdotal reports in the medical literature that Pycnogenol can help some children with ADHD, but a search of the medical literature does not reveal that formal studies of any of these supplements have been carried out. That doesn't mean that these supplements don't work; just that they haven't been studied. You can follow future studies of these supplements using a PubMed search (see Appendix C).

The following mail-order companies offer cheaper supplements than

---

*The herbs included were *Astragalus membranaceus, Codonopsis pilosula, Ligustrum lucidum, Lophatherum gracile,* and thread of ivory.

your local health-food store and their quality is excellent. You can call them for free catalogs:

Bronson: 1-800-235-3200
L & H Vitamins: 1-800-221-1152
SDV Vitamins: 1-800-738-8482

Here are some guidelines to follow when you give your child vitamins, minerals, and other supplements:

* Choose supplements that are not artificially colored and flavored and do not contain sugar. Also, some contain corn, which may bother the corn-sensitive child.
* Don't fall into the trap of thinking that by giving your child supplements you don't have to worry about his diet.
* Don't fall into the trap of thinking that if one tablet is good, ten would be even better.
* Some vitamins and minerals are toxic when taken in large amounts. These include vitamins A and D and the mineral selenium. Do not give more than the RDA of these.
* If your child is currently taking one or more supplements, give him a trial supplement-free period to make sure they are not contributing factors.
* Try multivitamin, multimineral, and herbal supplements separately for a week or so. If you try them all at once, you won't know what is helping or hurting.
* Discuss supplementation with your doctor to see if there are any reasons why your child should not take a particular supplement.

Giving your child certain vitamin, mineral, and other supplements may help him. Just keep in mind that providing an optimal diet, as described in Way 1, should be at the top of your priorities.

WAY 6.
SOLVE THE
YEAST CONNECTION

If your child has repeatedly taken antibiotics for ear or other infections, he may have a problem with an overgrowth of the intestinal yeast *Candida albicans*. When he takes antibiotics for an infection, the drugs kill both the bad and the good bacteria in his intestines. The good bacteria help keep the population of candida, normal inhabitants of the intestines, in check. When some of them are killed off, candida are allowed to thrive and multiply in the intestines, giving off toxins that affect the immune and nervous systems. Candida may also cause leakiness of the intestinal membranes, which leads to food sensitivities, a major problem for many children with ADD/ADHD.

Answer yes or no to the following questions related to yeast problems:

1. Was your child bothered by thrush as a baby?
2. Was he bothered by frequent or persistent diaper rashes?
3. Was he bothered by colic and irritability lasting over three months?

4. Are his symptoms worse on damp days or in damp, moldy places?

5. Are your child's symptoms better when snow covers the ground?

6. Has your child been bothered by recurrent or persistent athlete's foot or any other chronic fungal infections of his skin or nails?

7. Has your child taken antibiotics for recurrent ear infections?

8. Has your child had tubes surgically inserted in his ears?

9. Has your child been bothered by recurrent hives, eczema, or other chronic skin problems?

10. Has he received four or more courses of antibiotic drugs during the past year?

11. Has he received continuous (for a month or longer) antibiotic drugs?

12. If your child is a teenager, has he ever taken tetracycline for chronic acne?

13. Has your child taken prednisone or other cortisone-type drugs?

14. Has your child been bothered by persistent or recurrent digestive problems, including constipation, diarrhea, bloating, or excessive gas?

15. Does your child crave sugar?

16. Is your child's behavior worse after he eats sugary treats?

17. Does exposure to perfumes, insecticides, gas fumes, or other chemicals provoke symptoms?

18. Does tobacco smoke "turn your child on" or make him feel miserable?

The more questions to which you answered yes, the greater the chances that your child's behavior, allergies, and frequent ear and respiratory infections are yeast-connected.

Our world is populated by infinite numbers of tiny, microscopic organisms. They're found in the soil and on plants, vegetables, and fruits. One hundred trillion (give or take a few trillion) are also found all over and inside your child's body. These microorganisms include "good" bacteria, "bad" bacteria, molds, yeasts, and other tiny critters.

Many yeasts are beneficial. For example, we use baker's yeast to make bread rise and brewer's yeast to ferment fruit juices, sugar cane, and grains into alcohol. The common yeast *Candida albicans* normally lives on the skin and interior membranes of your child's body, including the mouth, esophagus, intestines, and vagina, and may cause minor infections of the mucous membranes of the mouth (thrush) and the moist areas around the rectum. Candida also causes vaginal yeast infections. Candida may be present at birth and colonizes most babies' bodies by four weeks of age.

When a child is healthy and his immune resistance is strong, candida cause no problems. But when your child receives repeated or prolonged courses of broad-spectrum antibiotic drugs—for example, amoxicillin; Septra Bactrim both consisting of (trimethoprim and sulfamethoxazole); Keflex (cephalexin); and other antibiotics commonly prescribed for young children troubled by repeated ear infections—yeast-related disorders may develop.

Although candida has long been known to be the cause of thrush (a yeast infection in the mouth) and vaginal yeast infections, only recently has it been recognized as a common cause of physical and mental symptoms. In 1961, allergist C. Orian Truss found that one of his patients who suffered from runny nose, migraine headaches, depression, and a vaginal yeast infection repeatedly experienced complete relief from all her symptoms when she received an injection of candida extract. Several years later, Dr. Truss tried this therapy with other patients and again achieved success. These patients experienced dramatic relief from a variety of unrelated mental and physical symptoms.[1]

Dr. Truss had this to say about candida in children:

> *The first clinical recognition of infection with* Candida albicans *often follows an infant's initial encounter with antibiotic. The infection may be respiratory—croup, tonsillitis, a cold, bronchitis, ear [infection], etc. After seven to ten days of a potent, yeast-stimulating antibiotic, yeast manifestations may appear. Oral thrush, diaper rash, and diarrhea are the most frequent.*
>
> *Unfortunately, after the use of the antibiotic has been discontinued, the previous state of health may not return. In addition to the symptoms induced by the yeast where it is growing on the skin and mucous membranes, there may be a clear nasal discharge not present previously. Restlessness, discontent, and irritability often accompany the "runny nose" and are responsible for*

the infant's inability to sleep restfully or without interruption for the normal duration. . . .

Chronic candidiasis is a very real problem in infants and children, interfering in many ways with normal growth and development and performance in school, predisposing them to allergic membranes and a vicious cycle of infections and antibiotics.[2]

Here's what may happen when your child takes antibiotics for an infection. Broad-spectrum antibiotics kill off friendly bacteria on the interior membranes of your child's body while they're killing the harmful bacteria. When this occurs, yeasts flourish and put out a toxin that affects various organs and systems in the body, including the immune system and the brain.[3] The yeast also damages the gut, making it "leaky," allowing large molecules from partially digested food to be absorbed into the bloodstream. The body reacts with an immune response to the invading foreign molecules. The result is multiple food allergies, which can lead to such symptoms as hyperactivity and attention deficits.

If your child's diet is rich in sugar and refined carbohydrates, it stimulates candida to grow and flourish. Candida love the sugar almost as much as your child does! You've probably added sugar to bread dough to feed the baker's yeast so it will reproduce. Eating sugar and refined carbohydrates feeds the yeast in your child's digestive tract, making the candida multiply and produce more toxins.

Your child's physical symptoms, hyperactivity, and behavior and learning problems may be related to toxins from candida and food allergies triggered by the increase of candida in the digestive tract. Yeast-connected behavior disorders should be suspected in any child who has received repeated or prolonged courses of broad-spectrum antibiotic drugs. And the diagnosis can be confirmed by the child's response to antifungal therapy.

Leo Galland, M.D., suggests that "a child who has had antibiotics more than once a year, who has *any type* of allergy, who has behavioral problems of any kind, or who develops behavioral problems *after* antibiotic treatment might have a yeast sensitization problem."[4]

Here's what one mother, Sarah, had to say about her hyperactive, irritable child.

Sally is seven years old. She is doing great now, but she used to be extremely hyperactive and irritable with severe temper tantrums that went on and on. Two nursery schools asked us to withdraw her from their school because of her behavior problems. We were devastated—expelled from nursery school! Sally was so hyperactive in kindergarten that she couldn't stay seated and rarely paid attention. She wasn't learning how to read or write. She was driving her teachers and family nuts with her behavior. Her nose was always stuffy and itchy. Sally continued to have ear infections and required a second set of tubes inserted in both ears.

Our doctor suggested we try Ritalin. It didn't help Sally's behavior, and it decreased her appetite. In the evening she was more hyperactive and had trouble falling asleep. Instead of trying other stimulant drugs, we decided to see a doctor here in town who had had success treating patients like Sally.

We saw our new doctor when Sally was six years old. The doctor was very interested in Sally's medical history. Sally had been a happy, "easy," baby. She was breast-fed and full of smiles and cooing. Then at six months, she came down with an ear infection and her pediatrician prescribed an antibiotic for ten days. She was okay for a few weeks, then she came down with another ear infection, which led to more, stronger antibiotics. She also developed a severe diaper rash and diarrhea. Her behavior began to change. Her sunny disposition disappeared. She cried nonstop. She was overactive always on the go, "wound up like a motor." I noticed every time she ate sugar, her behavior worsened, but her doctor assured me that sugar could not cause behavior problems. Her ear infections continued, and finally, when she was three, she had tubes surgically placed in her ears.

Our new doctor suspected that Sally had a chronic problem with yeast because of all the antibiotics she had received. He put Sally on a special sugar-free diet and prescribed the anti-yeast medication Nystatin. We also gave Sally supplements of "good" bacteria. Sally responded dramatically to the program. She looked better—healthy for the first time. Her nose stopped running. She could sit down to eat meals. The temper tantrums disappeared. We were so excited. So was her teacher, who found that Sally could now sit quietly and easily learned her lessons. Treating her yeast changed her life.

IDENTIFYING CHILDREN WITH
YEAST-RELATED ILLNESS

If your child's problems appear to be candida-related, a change in diet will help you determine whether or not yeast is the culprit.

First, have him avoid sugary foods, which promote yeast growth. Sugary foods and beverages include those sweetened with sucrose (table sugar), dextrose, fructose, honey, maple syrup, or malt syrups. Avoid fruit drinks, punches, and even 100 percent pure fruit juices. Limit fruit to two pieces a day that can be peeled and the peel discarded. Examples include oranges, tangerines, apples, pears, peaches, nectarines, pineapple, and melons. Avoid strawberries and similar unpeelable fruits because they have more mold and yeast on their surfaces. Fruit and fruit juices are rich in fruit sugar (fructose) and other carbohydrates that may promote yeast growth. Also, fruits are covered with yeasts. When juices are extracted yeast flourish by "eating" the natural sugar of the fruit juice. However, as your child improves, experiment with fruits and fresh-squeezed juices. If they don't cause symptoms, give them in moderation (no more than two servings of fruits a day).

Also avoid foods that contain yeast (as your child may be allergic to yeasts). These include bread, pastries, cheese, dried fruits, and some commercial soups. Avoid vinegar because it's a source of yeast. Also avoid vitamins that are not yeast-free. Malt is another yeasty product to avoid. Avoid mushrooms, a fungus related to yeast.

Is your child better on the yeast-elimination diet? After five to seven days, give him yeast tablets or yeasty foods to see if he shows a reaction. If his behavior deteriorates when he is eating yeasty foods, go back to the yeast-free diet for several months.

Your doctor may find a comprehensive digestive stool analysis helpful.* All it takes is a sample of your child's stool. This test gives your doctor all kinds of information. If there is a lot of yeast present, then you should follow the instructions in this chapter. However, for unknown reasons,

---

*Your doctor can order the comprehensive digestive stool analysis from Great Smokies Diagnostic Laboratory, 63 Zillicoa Street, Asheville, NC 28801-1074.

some children with a seeming yeast problem do not have an overgrowth of yeast but benefit greatly from antifungal therapy. This test will also help your doctor determine whether or not sufficient friendly bacteria, as well as damaging parasites, are present. The stool analysis also measures different indicators of digestion and absorption problems. For example, if meat and vegetable fibers are present, these would indicate that your child doesn't completely digest his food. A stool analysis may give your doctor all kinds of important information.

TREATING YEAST-RELATED ILLNESS

The goal of treating yeast-related illness is to weaken the candida and strengthen your child's immune system. To weaken the candida, keep your child on the yeast elimination diet. Give your child foods and supplements that help control candida overgrowth in his digestive tract. These include garlic and garlic products, and sugar-free yogurt with active cultures. Yogurt contains the friendly bacteria *Lactobacillus acidophilus*. Though, of course, if your child is sensitive to dairy products, you should avoid using yogurt. Powders and capsules containing friendly bacteria *Lactobacillus acidophilus* and *Lactobacillus bifidus* can be obtained from health-food stores and some pharmacies.

Think of giving your child acidophilus and bifidus in addition to yeast in terms of getting rid of weeds in your lawn. You could dig out the weeds or kill them with chemicals; however, if you did not replant with grass seed, there is a likelihood that the weeds would return. The treatment of a yeast problem involves both the suppression of yeast overgrowth and the reseeding of the intestines and vagina with normal organisms that can help prevent yeast growth.[5]

Avoid broad-spectrum antibiotics and cortisone-type drugs. Most fevers in children (perhaps 80 to 90 percent or more) are caused by viruses. Viral infections are usually "self-limiting." This means that your child's immune system conquers the infection without the help of medication. Current available antibiotics don't kill viruses. So don't twist your doctor's arm to prescribe antibiotics. Instead ask, "Is this antibiotic really necessary?"

Avoid high mold areas because molds are related to yeast and many people with yeast problems are also sensitive to mold. So keep your child out of piles of leaves and moldy attics and basements (Way 7).

Ask your doctor to prescribe an antifungal medication that helps eradicate or control yeast organisms in your child's digestive tract. Nystatin is the medication usually prescribed in patients with yeast-connected health problems. It is an antifungal drug that kills yeast but does not affect good bacteria and other germs. Nystatin is available in 500,000-unit oral tablets and as an oral suspension containing 100,000 units per milliliter. However, nutritionally oriented physicians usually prefer pure nystatin powder (*not* nystatin skin powder) manufactured by Lederle Laboratories because the liquid preparations contain sugar and are much more expensive than the powder. The tablets usually contain food coloring and other additives. If your child won't take the powder in water, try adding a couple of drops of liquid saccharin, or pack the powder into clear gelatin capsules. Dr. Crook maintains that most of his patients improve when they take 500,000 units (⅛ teaspoon of the powder) of nystatin four times a day. Occasionally, patients do well on a dose of ¹⁄₁₆ teaspoonful (or less) given four times a day. Some patients, Crook says, need to take nystatin for many months, until their immune and nervous systems return to normal.[6]

Nystatin is safer than most drugs physicians prescribe for their patients. It's virtually nontoxic and nonsensitizing and is well tolerated by infants and children, even with prolonged administration. It is safe because very little is absorbed from the intestinal tract.

Nevertheless, nystatin disagrees with some patients and may cause digestive symptoms or skin rashes. Some individuals develop other symptoms, including headache, fatigue, and flu-like symptoms or increased behavior problems, especially during the first few days of treatment. Just continue the medication and the other symptoms will stop.

If nystatin doesn't help your child, you could ask your doctor about another prescription drug, Diflucan (fluconazole), used to kill candida. It is more potent than nystatin and is absorbed from the intestines into the bloodstream.

Your doctor may declare that "yeast-related illness" is another fad diagnosis for children with ADHD and other health problems. She may refuse to prescribe nystatin. In this case, you can try over-the-counter products such as the fatty acid caprylic acid or grapefruit seed extract.[7] These natural, safe products kill yeast in the intestinal tract and help your child regain the balance between yeast and good bacteria. Start with a low dose and gradually increase the dosage until you reach the recommended dosage on the product label.

If your child has a "yeast problem," take the important steps to strengthen your child's immune system outlined in this chapter. Also, improve his diet (see Way 1), give essential fatty acids if indicated (see Way 4), and carefully choose vitamin and mineral supplements (see Way 5). All of these approaches can dramatically improve your child's behavior and health.

WAY 7.
IDENTIFY INHALANT
ALLERGIES

Thirty percent of Americans have a genetic predisposition for developing allergies. If your child is troubled by persistent or recurrent respiratory symptoms or ear problems, he may be sensitive to pollens, molds, house dust, or animal dander. (Allergies to foods can also cause nasal and respiratory symptoms.) Nasal allergy (allergic rhinitis) is the most common chronic disease, affecting 17 percent of Americans. The lining of the nose becomes inflamed by airborne allergens (dust, mold, pollen, and animal dander), causing symptoms in the nose, eyes, and throat. Sometimes it's difficult to tell the difference between colds and allergies. If a "cold" lasts more than seven days, symptoms are probably due to an allergy. Seasonal allergic rhinitis usually occurs in the spring and fall due to sensitivities to tree, grass, and ragweed pollens. Perennial allergic rhinitis occurs year round due to allergies to dust, mold, and pets. Allergic rhinitis can make your child feel irritable and cranky because he can't breathe well. When your child can't breathe properly, his brain orders adrenaline to be released, which makes children feel grumpy and ornery.

A child who has itching; sneezing; runny nose; itchy, watery eyes; and congestion that are not well controlled may act inattentive and experience learning problems during school hours.[1] At night, if a child is congested, he may experience sleep loss, which further affects his daytime fatigue and learning problems. These problems may occur in seasonal or perennial rhinitis. Moreover, some children experience sinus and middle ear infections and hearing loss. Many of the drugs used to treat allergic rhinitis cause problems in the central nervous system, leading to learning problems. If allergic rhinitis is a problem for your child and he is taking inhaled or oral medication to reduce the congestion, discuss side effects with your doctor. Newer drugs are less sedating and less likely to interfere with the central nervous system.

These airborne particles your child inhales may also directly make your child tired, irritable, and overactive. And in some children who aren't bothered by respiratory symptoms, inhalant allergies may cause other physical and behavior problems.

Linda commented about her two sons, Tommy and Jimmy:

Even though Tommy's nose often streamed and his eyes watered, I was surprised when testing for mold, dust, and pollens provoked dramatic behavior changes. He became anxious, irritable, hyperactive, and he also complained of a headache. On testing, Tommy showed a strong reaction to molds, dust, and ragweed and less serious reactions to tree and grass pollens. Treatment dramatically improved his behavior and respiratory symptoms. Today, Tom still sneezes and his nose still streams during ragweed season if the pollen counts are especially high, but he experiences no problems in attention or behavior.

I was amazed when Tommy's younger brother, Jimmy, reacted to molds, pollens, and dust with hostility and irritability. His legs also ached and he acted exhausted. Jimmy had never shown any typical respiratory allergies— no runny nose, sneezing, or asthma. Treating Jimmy for these inhalant sensitivities greatly improved his mood and behavior.

Answer yes or no to the following questions pertaining to your child's symptoms.

1. Is your child troubled by persistent or recurring respiratory problems such as chronic runny, stuffy, or itchy nose; sinusitis; ear infections, fluid in ears, or hearing loss; bronchitis; or asthma?
2. Do your child's symptoms occur year round but especially in the fall and winter months when the furnace constantly blows dust throughout the house?
3. Does your child feel or act worse when you vacuum or clean house?
4. Do your child's symptoms come on or get worse during the mold seasons in your area (usually the spring or fall months)?
5. Are your child's symptoms better during the winter if the ground is frozen and snow-covered?
6. Does damp, windy weather make his symptoms worse?
7. Does raking leaves, cutting grass, or digging in the dirt aggravate his symptoms?
8. Do your child's symptoms begin or get worse during your local pollen season?
9. Are they worse on days with the highest pollen counts?
10. Do his symptoms decrease or disappear with the first frost?
11. Are your child's symptoms aggravated by contact with a furry or feathered animal? Did his symptoms start or increase when you got a new pet?
12. During the pollen season, does your child feel better in an air-conditioned indoor setting than he does outdoors?
13. Does a hard, continuous rain bring relief during high-pollen months?
14. Are his symptoms worse on windy days during pollen season?

If you answered yes to one or more of these questions, you'll want to reduce your child's exposure to airborne particles. Following are some common airborne allergens your child should avoid.

HOUSE DUST

The fine gray powder that results from the natural deterioration of such household items as mattresses, carpeting, curtains, papers, books, and clothes; plus molds and pollens—that's house dust. Another component is the house-dust mite, a microscopic spider-like bug that is found wherever people are, especially in bedding and mattresses. Dust mites are the number-one cause of allergies because they produce highly allergenic feces and proteins. House dust is what you see floating, seemingly suspended, on sunbeams indoors. It's what you throw away when you empty your vacuum cleaner. Dust settles everywhere, and it accumulates in areas that aren't frequently cleaned. But even the best-kept houses have house dust in the air.

Here are ways you can reduce your child's exposure to house dust:

- Keep your child's bedroom as free of offending substances as possible. This will increase his tolerance to inhalant exposures during the rest of his day. Carefully clean the room at regular intervals. Don't use odorous chemicals (see Way 8).
- Remove any carpeting from your child's bedroom because it holds mold and dust particles. Avoid stuffed animals and other dust-collectors.
- Cover your child's mattress and pillow with an encasing that doesn't bother him. For example, Allercare makes hypoallergenic coverings for pillows and mattresses. (Avoid foam rubber or feather pillows, and odorous plastic encasings.)
- Change furnace filters frequently. New, more effective filters are now available from 3M, but they are more expensive. Installing an electronic air cleaner on your furnace may help, particularly if you also have your ducts cleaned professionally with special high-powered vacuums. Dust, molds, mildew, and bacteria love your air ducts. Your ducts are like a room that has never been cleaned!
- Clean and vacuum your house while your child is away. A vac-

uum with a hard, plastic body instead of a porous fabric will reduce the amount of dust you kick up while you vacuum. If you have an air cleaner on your furnace, run your furnace blower while you vacuum and for an hour afterward. This will remove 90 percent of the dust particles.

• Use a room air purifier in your child's bedroom and perhaps in other rooms in your house as well. (Holmes and Envirocaire are two brands widely available at reasonable prices.) Replace filters frequently.

• Leave doors open between rooms to maximize air flow inside and reduce dust and mold.

• At night, use nasal breathing correction strips to keep your child's nose open so he can breathe and sleep better.

MOLDS

Molds belong to the group of plants called fungi, which have no true leaves, stems, flowers, or green pigment and which reproduce by means of spores. You're probably familiar with the furry mold that grows on old bread or leftover food. There are thousands of different types of molds. They are found all over the world in soil, air, and water. They flourish in damp, dark areas, both inside and outside.

The weather affects the molds in the air you breathe. Rainfall, high humidity, and wind disperse mold spores, making the mold-sensitive child miserable. Molds tend to grow best in cool temperatures, without direct sunlight. Night air thus contains more spores than day. Although the air is never free of mold spores, in the winter when the ground is frozen and snow-covered, molds are less prevalent outdoors.

Molds are also present in certain foods, such as some cheeses. Persons who are mold-sensitive are frequently sensitive to other members of the fungi family—mushrooms and mushroom spores, baker's yeast, brewer's yeast (found in vinegar, B-vitamin preparations, and enriched foods).

Here are ways to reduce your child's mold exposure:

- Clean mold-prone areas frequently with tolerated disinfectants (borax, baking soda, or vinegar).
- Molds love every nook and cranny of your bathroom. They'll grow in your bathtub drain, on washcloths, damp towels, and in any crevice. Keep your bathrooms as dry as possible. Install a fan to keep the bathroom well ventilated. Scrub tiles and grout around tubs and showers with tolerated disinfectant.
- If your basement (especially one with a dirt floor) is damp, work to dry it out. Seal cracks in the walls or floor. Use a dehumidifier but be careful to keep it free of molds. Good ventilation and lighting also discourage dampness and molds.

ANIMAL DANDER

Any animal with fur or feathers can provoke allergic symptoms in sensitive children. Common culprits are cats, dogs, horses, rabbits, mice, hamsters, gerbils, parakeets, cattle, hogs, sheep, goats, and chickens. Unfortunately, short-haired animals are as allergenic as long-haired animals because the allergenic substances come from the saliva, urine, and dander (skin cells), not the fur itself. Animals that don't cause allergic reactions include snakes and turtles.

Here are some ways to reduce your child's exposure to animal dander:

- Keep Rover and Kitty out of the bedroom and outside if possible. If you don't own a pet, don't get one now.
- Give your pet a weekly bath. We did this with our cat—he was not pleased, but it seemed to help!
- Have your child wash his hands after he plays with his pet.
- Don't let your child empty the litter box.

POLLENS

Pollens are the yellow, powderlike particles found on flowers. They allow plants to reproduce. Heavy, sticky pollens are usually not a problem because they don't become airborne, but lighter pollens are easily carried by the wind, sometimes hundreds of miles. Fortunately, only a comparatively small number of these tend to be allergenic. The most common problem-causing pollens come from certain trees, grasses, and weeds. Ragweed is a well-known example.

The pollen season will depend on where you live. Your newspaper or TV and radio weather reports may give the pollen and mold counts for your area. These counts represent the number of grains of a specific pollen (usually ragweed) present in a given volume of air at a specified time and place. Follow these reports to help you correlate these pollens with your child's symptoms. Pollen seasons often overlap with high mold counts, but pollen-producing plants are killed by the first frost while high mold counts continue until snow or freezing temperatures arrive. You can also find out whether or not mold or pollen counts are high in your area by accessing CNN's home page: http://www.cnn.com/WEATHER/allergy/. Interestingly, children who are sensitive to ragweed are often allergic to watermelon, cantaloupe, and bananas.

One observant mother described her son's reactions to seasonal allergens:

I have a five-year-old son who was diagnosed with ADHD about a year and a half ago. He cannot take Ritalin or Dexedrine due to side effects, so his doctor placed him on hypertension medication, which he has been on for a little over a year. I have noticed that the last month or so his behavior has worsened tenfold with the increase in pollens in the air. He has been causing problems in the classroom, which is a first for him, for he is usually somewhat better at school than at home.

Here are suggestions for decreasing your child's exposure to pollens:

- Keep your child inside, particularly in the morning—pollen's peak time—close windows and doors, and use an air cleaner or air conditioner year round. Pollens are also higher on dry, windy days.

• Keep your car windows rolled up and use your car's air conditioner.

• Ideally, escape to the mountains or seashore, where pollen counts are much lower, during the worst weeks of your pollen season.

Should your child be tested and treated for inhalant allergies? The answer depends upon the severity and seasonal pattern of his symptoms. If he's bothered by troublesome respiratory symptoms—especially if they're seasonal—he should receive allergy skin testing and appropriate therapy. But don't be surprised if your allergist scoffs at the idea that treating inhalant allergies may improve behavior.

WAY 8.
IDENTIFY CHEMICAL
SENSITIVITIES

Toxic chemicals, such as insecticides, weed killers, diesel fumes, and petroleum-derived chemicals pollute our air, soil, food, and water and adversely affect our health. Natural gases, cleaning fluids, formaldehyde scents, tobacco smoke, and other chemicals may pollute your indoor air; in fact, indoor air can actually be more of a problem than outside air. These chemicals can make your child miserable. They can cause sneezing, coughing, asthma, aching muscles and joints, numbness, and other nervous system symptoms. What may surprise you is that chemicals may cause some children to be irritable, inattentive, spacey, aggressive, depressed, or hyperactive.

Does chemical exposure make *your* child feel sick, tired, nervous, depressed, irritable, spaced out, or hyperactive? Do chemicals "turn your child on"?

Answer yes or no to the following questions about your child and his exposure to toxic chemicals:

1. Has your child ever been exposed to massive amounts of toxic chemicals?
2. Is he frequently exposed to toxic chemicals at school, at home, or while pursuing hobbies?
3. Did his symptoms begin or worsen after moving to a new home, or going to a new school or one undergoing renovation?
4. Does your child seem more aware of chemical odors (particularly natural gas leaks) than other people are? Is he bothered by chemical odors that don't bother others?
5. Does your child crave the smell of certain chemicals?
6. Do you cook with gas, or do you heat your home with a gas floor-furnace, open gas heaters, or kerosene heaters?
7. If you cook with gas, does your child's behavior deteriorate when he's in the kitchen?
8. Is your child worse when he's riding in traffic, riding on a bus, or is in an area of high air pollution, or when you're pumping gas at a service station?
9. Does your child feel or act better in unpolluted places (in the country, in the mountains, or near the ocean)?
10. Does he show physical or behavioral symptoms when he is exposed to:
    a. A chlorinated swimming pool?
    b. Perfume and tobacco smoke at church or social gatherings?
    c. Chemical odors in a clothing or furniture store?
    d. Fresh paint?
    e. Pesticide sprays?
    f. Household chemicals?
    g. Recently manufactured plastics, such as a new shower curtain, lampshade, place mat, or car?
11. Does anyone smoke in your house or car?

If you answered yes to any of these questions, chemical sensitivity may play an important role in causing your child's health and behavior problems. You will need to play detective and observe your child while he is exposed to various chemicals. Keep a written diary of potential chemical troublemakers and how your child is acting and feeling. For example, one observant mother reports about her son's chemical sensitivities:

Jimmy is sensitive to many different chemicals. Some reactions are obvious; others are rather subtle. For example, as soon as Jimmy gets in a swimming pool that has chlorinated water, his nose streams so badly that everyone moves away from him! He sneezes over and over. When he gets out of the pool, he's irritable and depressed. Needless to say, he hates swimming, although he likes to go in the water at the lake. Exposure to fresh paint gives him a severe headache. Perfume and scented products make his nose run and he's more hyperactive. Jimmy loves the smell of gasoline. If allowed, he would like to get out of the car at the gas station and get a really good fix at the pump. Afterwards, he "bounces off the walls." Limiting Jimmy's exposures to these chemicals is really important to keep him healthy and calm.

If you suspect that your child is sensitive to various chemicals, you'll want to take steps to limit household chemicals so your child won't be breathing them in. Here are suggestions.

CLEANING CHEMICALS

If your child has inhalant allergies (see Way 7), you will want to keep your house as clean as possible. On the other hand, he may be sensitive to the cleaning products. Even if you do the cleaning while he's out of the house, the odors will linger. He may be sensitive to chlorine found in bleach, scrubbing cleansers, deodorizers, disinfectants, and swimming pools. He may also be sensitive to the ammonia found in glass cleaners, bathroom cleansers, and oven cleaners. Instead, you can use Bon Ami all-purpose cleaner, Arm & Hammer washing soda, Ivory soap, and pure castile soap. Borax or baking soda can substitute for powdered cleansers. Cut soap film from tiles and retard mold growth with vinegar. Shaklee's Basic H cleanser is often well tolerated and is suitable for many chores. To make your own glass cleaner, add 1 tablespoon vinegar to 1 quart water. Pour the mixture into a pump spray bottle. Avoid scented room deodorants. Choose unscented dishwasher detergents like unscented Electrasol, laundry detergents like unscented Tide, and unscented fabric softeners. If your child is sensitive to furniture polish, use Murphy's wood soap and 100 percent lemon oil or raw linseed oil on natural wood surfaces. Spot-test for safety first. Also, Earth Friendly Cleaning Products makes a line of household cleansers from all-natural ingredients.

COSMETICS, PERFUMES, AND OTHER PERSONAL-CARE PRODUCTS

Look for unscented products. You'll be able to find unscented deodorant, hair spray, and shaving cream. Choose unscented soaps, such as Basis or Almay. Don't use perfume or aftershave lotion until you know whether or not your child is chemically sensitive. The fragrance in shampoos can be a problem. You'll just have to try some out to see if they work for your child. For example, you could try Johnson's baby shampoo, Almay, and castile shampoo. Tom's of Maine, Nature's Gate, Desert Essence, Kiss My Face, Jason Natural, Aubrey, Natural Crystal, Better Botanicals, Clearly Natural, and Weleda are just a few of the companies that make natural, fragrance-free products.

Most toothpastes and mouthwashes are artificially colored. Look for a white toothpaste like Colgate's regular-flavor toothpaste (though it does contain saccharin and sorbitol), or natural toothpastes and mouthwashes like those made by Tom's of Maine, Desert Essence, Natural Tea Tree Oil, Natural Dentist, Nature's Gate, and Weleda.

DRUGS

If your child is sensitive to artificial colors and flavors, ask your doctor if there is an uncolored tablet that will do just as well. Colored coatings can be washed off in many cases, but ask your pharmacist or doctor first if this is okay—some coatings are necessary for the action of the tablet. Colored capsules can be emptied into clear gelatin ones supplied by your pharmacist. Most over-the-counter drugs for children—antihistamines, cough syrup, aspirin, Tylenol, and ibuprofen—contain artificial colors and flavors. Many contain sugar. Enlist your pharmacist's help in finding products your child can take.

FORMALDEHYDE

Particleboard shelves, furniture, and cabinets often contain formaldehyde. You can seal them well with paint or shellac. But keep them out of the house until the paint or shellac fumes dissipate completely. New carpeting often gives off fumes due to any present formaldehyde and petrochemicals, which may bother your child. Choose attractive, tolerated flooring (brick, hardwood, stone, terrazzo, cement, ceramic tiles, and some vinyl). Choose such adhesives as glues and tapes carefully. Prewash new fabrics and clothes before your child wears them, as they may be treated with formaldehyde. Stay away from homes with urea-formaldehyde foam insulation. Yellow fiberglass wrapped in aluminum is the best-tolerated insulation. Avoid all cosmetics and personal-care products that contain formaldehyde or Formalin.

NEWSPRINT, INKS, AND OFFICE SUPPLIES

Fresh newsprint may bother your child. Your child may also be sensitive to the inks in felt-tipped and ballpoint pens. Choose glues carefully. Many children are very sensitive to rubber cement and wood and airplane glue. Try to stick to the white school and stationery glues. Steer clear of scented paper.

PAINTS

Paint only in the spring and summer and leave the windows open as much as possible. You can also use an electronic air cleaner with a charcoal filter to absorb paint odors. Oil-based paints are usually more of a problem than water-based paints.

PESTICIDES

Remove all containers of pesticides, mothballs, and fly strips from the house. Use fly snatchers, mousetraps, and natural pest control methods to rid your house of pests. Orange Guard makes a pest control product that contains no inert chemicals or carcinogens; its main ingredient is orange peel extract. Keep your child indoors when your neighborhood is sprayed for mosquitoes and your neighbors' lawns are fertilized.

PETROLEUM PRODUCTS AND GAS FUMES

If you find that your child is chemically sensitive, you may want to replace gas stoves and furnaces and kerosene heaters with electric appliances. Fill up your car's gas tank when your child is not in the car. In traffic, keep your windows shut and don't drive too close to the vehicle in front of you, especially buses and trucks spewing strong gas fumes. If your child is calm before he leaves the house in the morning and becomes hyperactive and out of control on the school bus, the problem may be exhaust fumes from the bus seeping inside.

PLASTICS

Avoid soft, smelly plastics. For example, many shower curtains and window shades have a very strong vinyl smell when first taken out of the package. Air the curtain or shades in a closed-off room, the garage, or at the home of friends or relatives. New lampshades may also have the same plastic smell. Use shades made out of breathable fabrics.

TOBACCO

If you are a smoker or you have a smoker in the house, allow smoking outside only. Even so, the tobacco smoke will cling to your clothes and could bother your child. If you confine your smoking to one closed-off room, the fumes will get in the ventilation system and pollute your house. Never let anyone smoke in the family car. Always request seating in non-smoking sections of restaurants.

WATER

Your child should drink water free of chlorine, toxic chemicals, and lead. You can buy bottled water in glass jugs or locate an uncontaminated local spring or well. Store water in glass jugs. You may find it easier and cheaper to put a water filter on your cold water tap in the kitchen. Brita makes an excellent water filter. You just pour tap water into a large pitcher that contains a filter you replace periodically. Your family will really like the taste of pure water.

AVOIDING CHEMICAL EXPOSURE AT SCHOOL

Is your child's behavior a lot better at home, yet out of control at school? Is he better on weekends and during vacations? Are teachers and school personnel reporting unexplained symptoms such as headaches, runny noses, muscle pains, dizziness, and fatigue? It's possible your child's school building is part of the problem. Modern, airtight constructions often cause "sick-building syndrome." In an effort to conserve energy, buildings are sealed, and they recycle contaminated air. Air ducts may be dirty and circulate bacteria, mold, and dust. Air conditioners with inadequate filters may pollute the air with pollens, dust, and mold. Humidifiers may also encourage growth of molds and bacteria. Pests like cockroaches may inhabit your school. Their droppings are highly allergenic. In order to contain the roaches, toxic pesticides may be used regularly. Copy machines, fax machines, and laser printers give off chemical fumes. Cleaning chemicals may also contaminate the air. If your child is really sensitive to scents, his teacher's perfume or aftershave may bother him.

If your child is chemically sensitive, you'll need to work with his teacher and principal to reduce his exposure to chemicals that bother him. If he is sensitive to fragrances, after explaining the situation to his teacher, ask him or her not to wear aftershave, cologne, or perfume. If felt-tipped pens or glues and pastes bother your child, ask if you can provide him with alternate supplies that do not bother him. If new carpeting is going to be installed, ask if it is possible to lay the carpet during the summer months, when school is not in session. This same approach can be used with rooms that need to be painted. Try to develop a good rapport with your child's teacher and principal so that everyone can work together for the good of your child.

Jimmy's mother describes the problems her son experienced at school:

Chemical pollutants at school gave Jimmy really severe headaches. In fifth grade, the school hung new plastic curtains in all the classrooms. The vinyl smell was apparent to anyone who walked in the classrooms. He was also bothered by his teacher's perfume. It was embarrassing to ask his teachers not to wear perfume or aftershave, but they responded positively and were happy to help Jimmy. Approaching his peers was almost impossible.

We were blessed with caring, helpful school personnel from nursery school on. I enlisted their help by writing letters, initiating conferences, and loaning them appropriate books and articles. Not only did they cooperate in cleaning up the school environment, but they also helped the other children understand.

I hope your school personnel are cooperative. Try a low-key approach followed by profuse thanks and appreciation for their efforts.

•

Your child can't live in a bubble. The best you can do is reduce his exposure as much as possible and support his immune system as described in Way 5. Unfortunately, you will not be able to eliminate all the chemicals in your child's environment, but you can reduce the level of exposure, which can greatly help him.

WAY 9.
INVESTIGATE LEAD
AND ALUMINUM
POISONING

ADD and ADHD are thought to have a number of different biological "causes"—different causes for different children. Though lead poisoning is not the leading cause of ADD/ADHD, it can be a cause of the disorders and is devastating for the child who suffers from it. Children with and without ADD/ADHD who have lead poisoning need to be identified and treated.

Does your child suffer from any of the following?

- Short attention span
- Hyperactivity
- Learning disabilities
- Slow development
- Decreased growth
- Impaired hearing
- Brain damage

- Stomachaches or headaches
- Poor appetite
- Sleep problems
- Irritability, fatigue, or restlessness

Although your child may appear healthy, even low levels of lead in his blood may cause serious problems. Surprisingly, a child may be experiencing lead poisoning and not feel sick. Lead is a toxic mineral that substitutes for essential minerals such as calcium, iron, and zinc in the body, so the presence of lead disturbs a number of important physiological reactions that depend on these minerals. Lead interferes with the development and functioning of all body organs, especially the kidneys, red blood cells, and the central nervous system.

Lead poisoning was once thought to be a problem only in children from poorer neighborhoods, but now it's recognized that families who live in older houses or apartments may also be at risk. In the United States more than 3 million children—one out of every six children age six and younger—have toxic levels of lead in their bodies.

The Centers for Disease Control recommends that all children be screened for lead in the bloodstream at age one and that older children be checked every couple of years. Certainly, if your child is experiencing any of the above problems, you will want to ask your pediatrician about measuring lead levels right away. Your child's blood lead concentration should be under 10 micrograms per deciliter. If your child's blood level is between 10 and 19 mcg/dl, he has mild lead poisoning. If your child's blood level is between 20 and 44 mcg/dl, your child has moderate lead poisoning. A level between 45 and 69 mcg/dl indicates severe lead poisoning, and anything over 70, of course, is a medical emergency. Even in children with lead levels as low as 10, IQ scores are lower, development is slower, and attention problems are apparent. Some children with low blood levels of lead can exhibit serious symptoms that improve when they and their environments are treated. Some children with high levels have minor symptoms. Regardless of the number of symptoms exhibited, if there is lead in your child's bloodstream, he needs appropriate medical treatment.

Your child can be exposed to lead in any number of ways. Most houses built before 1960 contain leaded paint, and houses built as recently as 1978 may even contain leaded paint. Young children like to put things they find in their mouth. This is a common way for children to be exposed to lead, as many things could be lead-based, particularly small paint chips or even dirt. Even when people determine that the paint used in their home is lead-based and try to do the right thing by having it removed, there can be problems. As the paint is removed or during other types of remodeling, small lead particles can be released into the air, and if the child is around, he will inhale these particles. Water may pick up lead particles if the pipes are soldered with lead. Testing your water is inexpensive—$15 to $25. Some pottery is lead-based or decorated with lead-based paint. If your child eats foods that were held in such pottery, he will be ingesting lead. Don't let him eat foods that have been stored in pottery containing lead.

HELPING CHILDREN WITH LEAD POISONING

If your child has an elevated lead blood level, you'll want to work closely with your doctor to reduce the levels. First, if lead levels are high, you'll want to discuss the possibility of using nontoxic chelating drugs such as succimer to lower lead levels. Second, you'll want to identify and drastically reduce the sources of lead in your child's environment (see above). Third, eating right is important, too. Children who consume enough zinc, calcium, and iron absorb less lead. Adopting a healthy diet as described in Way 1 will help your child get rid of the lead in his body. Fourth, nutritional supplements are important. Sidney M. Baker, M.D., formerly of the Gesell Institute, recommends the following nutritional supplements:[1]

- Elemental zinc, 15 to 60 milligrams daily
- Calcium, 1 to 2 grams (1,000 to 2,000 milligrams) daily.
  Avoid calcium supplements derived from dolomite or bone
  meal as these may be contaminated with lead.
- Magnesium glycinate, 100 to 300 milligrams daily
- Selenium, 50 to 200 micrograms daily
- Vitamin B6, 50 to 200 milligrams daily

- Vitamin C, 1,000 to 4,000 milligrams daily. If this dose causes loose stools, reduce the dose by half.
- Reduced glutathione, 250 to 750 milligrams daily
- Acetyl cysteine, 500 to 1,500 milligrams daily

OTHER SOURCES OF INFORMATION ABOUT LEAD

For more information about lead poisoning you can call 1-800-LEAD-FYI, an information center set up by the Environmental Protection Agency. The center will send you a packet of information about lead poisoning in children and how to safely remove lead from your child's environment. You can also find informative home pages on the Internet. Interesting home pages include:

- "HomeSafe" at www.leadpro.com. This website has helpful information about sources of lead poisoning, how to test for lead, and how to prevent future exposure. To find a certified inspector or contractor trained in removing lead call 1-800-648-LEAD.
- "ParentsPlace.com." This website has all kinds of helpful information for parents. To access the lead poisoning information, search for "lead poisoning."

Lead poisoning is probably *not* the cause of your child's problems, but it's easy and inexpensive to rule out. As Dr. Baker has emphasized: "Lead is the most abundant poison in the environment and should always be considered when a child has a behavior problem even if exposure to this substance is not likely."[2]

ALUMINUM

Like lead, aluminum is a toxic heavy metal that doesn't belong in your child's body. Elevated plasma aluminum levels in children have been associated with ADHD and learning disabilities. Simple analyses will determine whether or not your child is suffering from aluminum toxicity, as aluminum levels can be measured in hair, blood, and urine. Cooking foods, especially acidic ones like tomato sauce, in aluminum pots releases the aluminum into the foods. Instead, use cast iron, glass, porcelain, or stainless steel cookware. I've noticed that covering some foods—cooked rice, for example—with aluminum foil leads to the transfer of small specks of aluminum to the foods. So if you're going to use foil, wrap the food in waxed paper, then the foil. Avoid baking powder that contains sodium aluminum sulfate. Rumford is an aluminum-free brand you can find at your health-food store. Aluminum can also be taken into the body through antiperspirants, toothpastes, antacids, and municipal water supplies. Aluminum-free products can be found at your health-food store. Make sure your child takes care to drink only purified water.

Heavy-metal poisoning is probably not the cause of your child's ADD/ADHD symptoms. Nevertheless, it is important to rule this out as a possibility, as it is a significant factor for those children who suffer from it.

WAY 10.
ENHANCE
PERCEPTION

Perception is a daily part of our lives. Our brains are constantly receiving messages that they must process in order for us to make sense of our environment. Additionally, we must "see" in order to read, do math, take tests, do homework, copy, and write. But Jeff, who is in sixth grade, is having trouble in school. He cannot sit still while doing homework and is easily distracted. His teachers want him evaluated for ADD or ADHD. His mother feels that medication is not the answer. He does not complete assignments. He avoids reading and does not do as well as he could on tests. He is a bright, verbal child who does not appear to have a learning disability. He may be acting out because he is having a specific type of learning problem called scotopic sensitivity/Irlen syndrome.

Answer yes or no to the following questions regarding your child's perception:

1. Does your child skip words or lines when reading?
2. Does your child reread lines?
3. Does your child lose his place while reading?
4. Is your child easily distracted when reading?
5. Does your child need to take breaks from reading often?
6. Does your child find it harder to read the longer he reads?
7. Does your child get headaches when he reads?
8. Do your child's eyes get red and watery when he is reading?
9. Does reading make your child tired?
10. Does your child blink and squint while reading?
11. Does your child prefer to read in dim light?
12. Does your child read close to the page?
13. Does your child use his finger or other markers to help him read?
14. Does your child get restless, active, or fidgety when reading?

If you answered yes to three or more of the above questions, then your child may have scotopic sensitivity/Irlen syndrome, or SSS. This is not a visual problem. The eyes themselves are not the source of the problem, and routine eye screenings and exams will not pick up SSS; nor can optometrists or ophthalmologists correct this problem. Psychological and educational evaluations are not helpful, either. Instead, the problem is a perceptual dysfunction in the brain due to sensitivity to certain colors or wavelengths of light. Individuals with SSS may be sensitive to glare, brightness, and certain lighting. SSS occurs on a continuum and is more severe in some people than others. A few people with less severe SSS can excel at reading in school by working extra diligently.

Helping a child with poor reading is like trying to solve a jigsaw puzzle. You have to identify the correct pieces, put them together, and solve the puzzle. For some readers, identifying and correcting SSS may be a major solution, for others it may be only one of several factors, and for some children with reading problems there are no signs of SSS. SSS has a genetic component. Eighty-four percent of children with SSS have one or both parents with the disorder, so it would be helpful to know whether the parents have SSS.[1] Both parents should answer the following questions:

1. Do you build breaks into reading?
2. Do you prefer reading newspapers or magazines to books?
3. Do you get eyestrain or fatigue, tired, or even headaches if you read too long?
4. Do you find it harder to read under fluorescent lights?
5. As a child, were you told to stop reading in dim lighting?
6. Do you find it harder to read material on high-gloss white paper?
7. Do words seem to move, blur, or come together when reading?
8. Does the background of a page seem bright when you read?
9. Does the white background make patterns or look like rivers running down the page?
10. Do you reread passages for comprehension?
11. Are you a slow reader?
12. Are you an inefficient reader?
13. Do you find continuous reading difficult?

If you answered yes to any of those questions, you may be thinking, "Wow, no one has ever asked me those questions before. They describe my reading problems to a T." Here's how one adult described his reading problems:

The letters have a life of their own. The print is not black but unevenly shaded, and the background is glaring. The words I try to read are not firmly printed on the page but seem engaged in a complex dance, and other words keep crowding in.

There are flashing lights blocking things out. Flashing red blobs obliterate the page. The print disappears, and assorted colored shapes drift over the page. Reading is harrowing.[2]

Many children with SSS struggle in school. Teachers and parents may accuse the child of not trying hard enough. They don't understand the child's behavior in class. Here's what one girl, Susan, had to say about her school problems:

My parents told me I was a very bright little girl and my only problem was not being able to read from left to right. I thought I was retarded. As I grew older, school became a frightening experience. I was in regular classes. And I wanted to do well. I didn't want people to make fun of me. My younger brother was doing well in school. My parents were proud of him, and I wanted them to be proud of me, too. I began to live in a make-believe world where my school problems didn't exist. If I didn't get the grade I wanted, I would lose the paper or doctor up the grade. I didn't want the teachers to discover that I couldn't do the work, so I would cut classes, go to the library, or sit on the lawn. My teachers would tell me I needed to work harder. My parents were told that I could do better if I paid attention in class.

I often thought, why can't I read like other kids? If I promise to work very hard, will you make me like the other kids?[3]

DISCOVERY OF SCOTOPIC SENSITIVITY SYNDROME

How did researchers discover that certain poor readers have perception problems? In 1981, the federal government established a program at California State University at Long Beach to study adults with reading disabilities. Helen Irlen was chosen to coordinate the program. Over a period of eighteen months, Helen Irlen and her coworkers interviewed more than 1,500 adults about their reading problems. One subgroup emerged. Although this group was adequate in their decoding skills, phonetic skills, and sight vocabulary, they struggled with reading. Here are some of things the adults told Irlen:

- "Reading is unpleasant. I become restless and fidgety."
- "I find that I fall asleep from reading."
- "I hate to read because I have to read something three or four times to comprehend it."
- "No matter what I do, I read slower than anyone around me.

When everyone else finishes a chapter, I still might be on the
first or second page."

- "I can't look at the page for very long. I have to keep putting
it down."[4]

Irlen proceeded to interview both proficient readers and those who
struggled to read. When asked to describe what they saw, proficient readers
said they saw words and letters. But some of those who struggled with
reading saw words that ran together, words that turned into black lines,
and other distortions. Irlen chose thirty-five adult problem readers. Over
the next nine months, these adults visited all kinds of professionals to evaluate and treat their problems. None made any significant differences in
taming the distortions. One day Irlen was working with a group of five
students. One student had with her a red overlay she had used previously
for vision training exercises. Another student picked it up and placed the
overlay on what she was reading.

Lo and behold, the distortions disappeared and the letters stopped sway-
ing back and forth! But the other students did not experience the same
improvement with the red overlay. Many different colored overlays were
tried on all the students. Of thirty-five students with visual perception
problems, thirty-one were helped by the color overlays. Irlen found that
different students improved with different colors and that each student had
a color that was best for him.

While the colored overlays greatly helped the students, they complained
that they were cumbersome, and fluorescent lighting still bothered them.
So the research progressed to the use of colored lenses in glass frames.
What's even more exciting is that now specially tinted contact lenses are
available to treat SSS. They are clear contact lenses except for the area that
covers the pupil (the black of the eye). The centers of the lenses are tinted
with your child's best reading color. Because the color is only over the
pupil, they are invisible—they do not change the color of his irises. They
can be worn all the time, and no one can tell.

EFFECTS OF SSS

Does your child behave better at home, where the lighting is dimmer and there are no fluorescent lights? Is his behavior worse at school or in certain stores when he's under fluorescent lights? The majority of the population is not bothered by fluorescent lights or bright lights. But individuals with SSS may have a difficult time under bright lights or fluorescent lights. Picture your child sitting in class under bright fluorescent lights. After a few minutes of reading or listening, he becomes quite uncomfortable. He may get a headache, feel exhausted, fidget and squirm in his seat, become aggressive, or feel sick to his stomach. He can no longer pay attention so he gets up and moves around the room and talks with his friends. Of course, then he's in the doghouse with his teacher, who says, "Why can't you sit still? You're supposed to stay in your seat. Why aren't you reading your textbook? You could do better if you would only try harder." Finally he gets referred to the school study team, which recommends he be placed on Ritalin. The child doesn't understand why he is so fidgety and inattentive. He assumes that things look the same for all the other children. The child is made to feel that he is "bad" and even "stupid." His self-esteem plummets. No one stops to ask him, "How do you feel when you sit in class, and how does it feel when you read?" One seventeen-year-old who had been suspended from school answered, "My eyes feel like they're being squeezed together, my head feels like it's in a vise. Then I start to get a severe headache, my stomach feels queasy, and I experience a cold sweat." It's no wonder this student hated school, couldn't do the work, acted out, and was labeled disruptive.

The teacher does not understand that the classroom itself is causing this student to be inattentive and impulsive and is interfering with his behavior and learning ability. First, the fluorescent lights may cause environmental distortions. The teacher may seem to be moving even if she is not. Or she may have a glow around her, all of which becomes distracting and affects listening. In newer schools, windows have been eliminated or downsized for security purposes, so there is little natural light for the student to read by. Second, the bright, shiny white pages of the book contribute to the child's discomfort—the letters, words, and lines can seem to jump around and not make any sense. Third, certain bright or fluorescent colored papers affect the child and add to his problems. Stripes, polka dots, plaids, or bright colored papers on the walls are common culprits. Usually bright, fluorescent colors such as shades of orange, goldenrod, and other bright yellows are problems for the child with SSS. Fourth, the floor pattern is important, too. If the carpeting is a bright color or maybe black-and-white tiles, it may add to the problem. Blackboards or green chalkboards are often replaced with "white" boards. They are bright white and shiny. Copying from these boards becomes a frustrating, futile effort for the child with SSS. It's no wonder that his attention span is short.

SSS can affect an individual in more areas than reading. Writing or drawing on white paper is equally frustrating. Handwriting may be illegible with unequal spacing or letter size. Math is a nightmare because the columns don't line up properly. Music is another major problem with all the lines, notes, and special symbols. Children with SSS who like music and take piano lessons learn by watching their teacher's hands and listening to the tune, then trying to replicate it. Sight-reading is next to impossible. The child suffers not only academically, but also at sports. Children with SSS are often clumsy. No matter how much they practice, it's very difficult for them to judge the distance to the ball in baseball or to hit the ball with a bat. No matter how hard they try, children with SSS are often unsuccessful in school and extracurricular activities. Their self-esteem is often at rock bottom.

THE EFFECTIVENESS OF IRLEN COLORED LENSES

Various studies have supported the Irlen method of diagnosing and treating SSS.[5] In one study, teachers selected 105 children who were reading at at least eighteen months below their grade level.[6] All 105 children were screened for SSS. Sixty-seven were considered "scotopic" and twenty-five "non-scotopic." During the screening, the best color transparency was chosen on an individual basis. Every child who was given the correct color overlay experienced improvement in reading rate, sixteen of seventeen improved in reading accuracy, and all improved in reading comprehension.

The results were highly significant when these children were compared with other groups of scotopic children who were given clear overlays and those who were given incorrect colors.

A study by the New York City schools looked at twenty-six children experiencing academic/reading problems who also had SSS.[7] During a four-month period, half the students used a colored overlay during reading instruction while the other half did not. Those who used the colored overlays during reading instruction made statistically significant gains in passage comprehension, word identification, and reading accuracy. Those students who received the same reading instruction without colored overlays made no advances in any of the areas tested.

In another study, thirty-nine learning-disabled high school students were screened for SSS.[8] Fifty-six percent showed moderate to severe perceptual problems and were given colored overlays. The students were tested again after five months. Results showed that those who used their colored overlays made the greatest gain, and those who did not use them lost six months in reading comprehension.

GETTING HELP FOR YOUR CHILD

Suppose you suspect after you read this chapter that your child has SSS. What can you do? First, read Helen Irlen's *Reading by the Colors*. Next, contact the Irlen Institute at 5380 Village Road, Long Beach, CA 90808, or by telephone at 1-562-496-2550. The staff will be able to tell you where your nearest screener is. At the screening, you and your child will answer many questions about home, school, and work environments. Taking a family history is an important part of the screening process because of the genetic component of SSS. Parents sit in on screenings. This is important for several reasons. First, you may identify other family members with SSS. Second, you will get a better idea of your child's distorted environment and how he feels about it. Third, you may try some of the screening tasks yourself. If you have trouble with the tasks, your child may feel comforted to know he's not the only one. Finally, various colored overlays are systematically tried to see which one works best. You will see how colored lenses will help your child. Next, if your child shows signs of SSS that improve with color overlays, you will be referred to the nearest clinic. Irlen colored lenses will be selected for your child. Remember, they will not be the same color as the overlay. There are screeners and clinics throughout the world. A simple screening, which determines whether or not a client has SSS, is $45. A more complete diagnostic examination, which includes the determination of the client's appropriate-colored filters, runs under $500. The tinting of lenses costs about $45. All Irlen clinics offer the colored contact lenses.

If your child has reading problems due to SSS, he may still have some reading problems to overcome. Irlen comments: "The use of colored overlays, filters, or other aids as treatment for Scotopic Sensitivity Syndrome is not meant to replace reading remediation. Rather, the purpose is to eliminate the perceptual problems that inhibit the learning process. SSS might be only one of several layers contributing to reading problems."[9]

SSS AND ADD/ADHD

In Helen Irlen's experience, up to one-third of children with ADD or ADHD have SSS as a large piece of their attention problem.[10] These children are inattentive because they're distracted by their environment as they perceive it. They are impulsive and act out because they're frustrated with themselves and the class and books they don't understand. They may be overactive because they can't stand to sit still, and moving around helps them make order out of their environment. Irlen has found that some children with ADD or ADHD are able to stop their stimulant medications while others can reduce the dose.

In the 1970s, researchers John Ott and Lewis Mayron studied children in classrooms. Using time-lapse photography, they taped hyperactive children in a classroom with fluorescent lights. The children were out of their seats and "climbing the walls." Next, the children were taped in a classroom lit with full-spectrum lights. The children were calm and quiet.[11]

•

As Irlen says, "No child wants to be bad, no child wants to be stupid, no child wants to do poorly in school. Adults must look for the causes of the child's behavior. Too often educators and other professionals declare that they cannot find any reason why a child is having problems so therefore the child should just try harder. Self-esteem lasts a lifetime. We should be working to find new ways to help children."[12]

WAY 11.
CONSIDER
CRAWLING LESSONS

When your child was a baby, you probably watched in wonder as he crawled and learned to explore his world. Yet the importance of a baby's crawling lies not just in increasing his locomotion, but also in the maturation of one of his reflexes. The maturation of this reflex is necessary in order for him to have later success in school, at home, and even in sports.

Answer yes or no to the following questions about your child:

1. a. Did your child skip the crawling stage, or did he crawl in a strange way?
   b. Did your child crawl for only a short period of time—fewer than six months?
   c. Did your child walk early—before age one?
   d. Did your child spend a lot of time in playpens or walkers?
   e. Did your child wear leg braces or casts during the crawling stage?
2. Does your child have difficulty sitting still in the "proper" position?

    a. Does he stand up after sitting for a while, even though he is in a situation in which he knows he should remain seated, such as in school or church?

    b. Does he fidget?

    c. Does he slouch?

    d. Does he wrap his feet around the chair legs?

    e. Does he sit on one foot, lie down, or change position frequently?

3. Does your child have difficulty writing?

    a. Does he write laboriously?

    b. Does he write sloppily?

    c. Does he write very small or very large?

    d. Does he break pencil points frequently?

    e. Does he try to stand up to write?

    f. Does he avoid writing?

    g. Does he lose his place frequently when copying work from the chalkboard or a book?

4. Does your child have difficulty with his sense of direction?

    a. Does he confuse left and right?

    b. Does he need extra time or a "marker" to determine left from right?

    c. Does he read and/or write "backwards"?

5. Does your child have problems with coordination?

    a. Is he clumsy or poorly coordinated?

    b. Does he have trouble with skipping, marching, running and catching, or running and throwing?

    c. Does he avoid certain sports or certain positions in sports?

    d. Does he prefer swimming underwater or doing the breaststroke or the butterfly stroke to swimming freestyle?

6. Does your child have difficulty with homework?

    a. Does he avoid or postpone the beginning of homework?

    b. Does he take an extra long time to complete homework?

    c. Does he rush through homework?

    d. Does he often not finish homework?

7. Does your child have difficulty maintaining attention?

    a. Does he have trouble focusing on a task and staying with it?

    b. Does he daydream?

    c. Is he easily distracted?

    d. Does he "fiddle" with everything on his desk?

If you answered yes to three or more of these questions, especially the questions about crawling, your child may have an immature symmetric tonic neck reflex, or STNR. "Symmetric" refers to both sides of the body working together; "tonic" refers to a change in muscle tension or tone; and the neck reflex is an automatic response activated by changes in the neck position. So STNR is a normal reflex that occurs when the arms, neck, and head move in opposition to the legs. You may be familiar with other reflexes that a baby is born with or develops early in life. For example, the sucking reflex is present at birth and continues for six months. The sneezing reflex is also present at birth but continues throughout a lifetime. A baby is not born with STNR but develops this reflex at four to eight months, when the neck, arms, and legs automatically move together. At around six months of age, a baby first begins to adopt the "cat" position, sitting back on his legs with his head up and his arms straight down to the floor in front of him. Next, the baby learns to rock back and forth. Finally, this motion leads to one hand reaching out, and the baby learns to crawl. As the baby grows older and his normal motor development occurs, his STNR is less in control. The child should crawl correctly for at least six months to suppress the STNR. If he did not crawl for at least six months, the STNR will not have the opportunity to mature and will continue to affect the child's movement long after it no longer should. By the age of two, the baby should be in control of his body and the STNR should be diminished.

What is incorrect crawling? Here are examples. Some babies crawl backwards. Other babies stick their rears up in the air, preventing their knees from touching the ground, while keeping their hands and feet on the floor. Some children crawl with their bellies on the floor like soldiers in the army. Other children roll instead of crawl. They may become so proficient at rolling that they can roll around corners! Some children scoot across the floor. Other children "frog jump" instead of crawling correctly. None of these crawling techniques helps mature the STNR.

There may be environmental factors that influence how much time a baby spends crawling. The baby may have worn leg braces to correct physical defects. A child who spends a lot of time in a playpen might not get enough crawling time. A child who is placed in a walker doesn't have the opportunity to crawl. A child needs to crawl normally and for at least six months.

A child (or adult) with an immature STNR will have trouble sitting comfortably. When he tries to sit still, he feels physically miserable. This is because the STNR is still present, pulling the top part of the body in one direction and pulling the lower part the other way. The good news is that the STNR can be matured in children and adults through special crawling exercises.

PROBLEMS AT SCHOOL

The child with an immature STNR may have a very hard time sitting in school. Teachers are constantly telling their students to sit still and listen and to sit up straight. I bet you remember that from school. I can just hear my sixth grade teacher telling us all to sit up straight so we could learn better. But a child with an immature STNR is very uncomfortable in this position—legs bent, head up, and arms bent. Instead, he is more comfortable if the top part of his body is doing the opposite of what the lower part does. These children may be able to sit normally and quietly, but not for long periods of time and not comfortably.

His teacher may have commented:

- "Why can't Johnny sit still?"
- "I spend half my time just trying to keep Johnny in his seat."
- "The work Johnny does is good, but I have to keep after him all the time to get him to finish it."
- "The poor kid has missed three recesses this week trying to get all the work done."
- "He squirms around so much he misses half the directions."
- "If Johnny would just try a little harder . . ."[1]

Children with STNR are so uncomfortable in school they devise coping mechanisms in order to feel more comfortable. Some children, the "reachers," sit at their desks with their arms stretched out in front of them on the desk. With their arms straight, they can be more comfortable writing while their legs are bent. If they reach far enough in front of them, however, they irritate the person in front of them and get into trouble. Some children, the "slouchers," sit in the normal writing position but extend their legs out straight. They may put their feet on the desk in front of them and again annoy their neighbor and teacher. Then there are the "chair tippers." These children will tip the chair back so that their legs are out straight. The "foot lockers" wrap their legs around the chair legs and lock them in place. This helps the child sit still. Other children may sit on one or both legs in an effort to get comfortable. Then there are the "head resters," who put their heads down on their arms to write. The "standers" are children who feel much more comfortable standing up. The "squirmers" are children who aren't allowed to assume the above positions, so they squirm all day long. You can imagine how thrilled teachers are with all these children.

Here's the story Nancy O'Dell, Ph.D., and Patricia Cook, Ph.D., tell about a child, Beth, who couldn't sit still while being tested.

One little girl, Beth, did very poorly on a listening test we gave her. Even though she was seated during the testing, her feet were in constant motion. We suspected that Beth's antsiness and the noise she herself was making contributed to her low score on the test. We allowed Beth to stand, which she did quietly, and gave her another form of the test. Under these conditions, Beth scored much better on the listening test. Her basic listening problem was self-distracting noise and motion, rather than a hearing loss. She was doing poorly in listening because she was doing so poorly in sitting quietly.[2]

Children who squirm and can't sit comfortably are often labeled as having ADHD. Drs. Cook and O'Dell have found that at least 75 percent of the children they see with ADHD have an immature STNR. These children may act like yo-yos—up and down, up and down in their seats.

They make frequent trips to the pencil sharpener, to the water fountain, or to the bathroom. They may jiggle their legs constantly. They have to move something, so they'll tap their pencils, disrupting everyone around them. Or they'll take a pen and click the cap on and off repeatedly. They may move their mouths and jabber constantly until everyone wants to tell them to shut up! But this is how these children cope with the discomfort of sitting still.

Children with an immature STNR often struggle to write well. Their papers are often messy and half-finished. Other children with STNR may produce beautiful papers, but it may take them much longer compared to the other students. They may stay in during the lunch period or recess to finish their work. Drs. Cook and O'Dell estimate that writing is ten times harder for children with an immature STNR. Naturally, as they continue to fail, their self-esteem goes down. They decide, "Why should I try? I'm just going to get an F." Or they'll say, "I don't care about school. It's dumb." So these children conclude, "Why bother?"

PROBLEMS AT HOME

At home, STNR children are often disruptive. Parents must have the patience of saints to deal with these children day in and day out. Perhaps you have made the following comments to your child:

- "Why can't you sit up at the dinner table?"
- "How many times do I have to tell you not to sit on your legs?"
- "Don't do your homework lying on the floor. Why do you think we bought you a desk?"
- "We just can't take you to church anymore. You're all over the pew."
- "You just don't try hard enough!"[3]

Homework is a common source of frustration for the whole family. One father commented:

I've been doing the exercises with my nine-year-old daughter, who has had learning problems at school. It used to take her forever to complete her assignments. She would come home from school and start her homework immediately and still have to work on it for several hours after dinner. She and I did the crawling exercises together. Now she finishes her homework in no time at all and can go out and play and be a child! We're even able to play Frisbee. Before she did the exercises she could not catch the Frisbee.[4]

Mealtime is another common problem for families with children with STNR problems. They can't sit. They jump up and down. They may talk constantly. At the end of the meal everyone is in a bad mood. For example, Billy had an immature STNR and learning problems. Billy had started to walk very early, after crawling for no longer than several weeks.

Billy was squirming to the point of being disruptive. His mother commented that even their family meals were disrupted because Billy was in constant motion. Dinner conversations were interrupted by "Sit down, Billy," "Sit up straight, Billy," "Billy, stop swinging your legs; you're kicking your sister," and on and on.[5]

HELPING YOUR CHILD

If your child appears to have an immature STNR, you'll want to get O'Dell and Cook's book *Stopping Hyperactivity*. Your bookstore or library can order it for you if it isn't on the shelves. This book will describe the crawling exercises for you in detail, with accompanying photographs. The authors have also produced an outstanding educational videotape that demonstrates how to do the crawling exercises correctly. The exercise program takes fifteen minutes a day, five days a week, for about six months. The child must be five years or older. Once "fixed," the reflex problem is cured for life.

In the meantime, here are a few ways to work around the STNR problem.

At School

Ask your child's teacher to allow him freedom to choose how to sit. He'll feel more comfortable and accomplish more work. Also ask the teacher if the child could use a word processor to do work more often, allowing the child to write less. Your child will probably be more comfortable doing work this way. Be patient!

At Home

Allow your child more freedom to sit as he pleases. Eating dinner while standing up with one leg bent on the chair will make your child more comfortable. Let the child choose how he wants to sit while doing his homework. Using pencil "cushions" that fit over pens or pencils will relax your child's grip and make writing much easier. Understand that making the bed and hanging up clothes are difficult jobs for these children. I am not saying that you should exempt your child from these chores—just be understanding. Allow him some leeway in how he goes about getting those chores done and the amount of time it takes him to get them done. A lower rod in the closet will help your child hang up his clothes much more easily.

Sports

Your child may have avoided playing sports because he's poorly coordinated. Baseball and basketball are probably especially frustrating. But playing on the line in football might work out, whereas being the quarterback isn't realistic. Wrestling or running track may work out well. Soccer is another sport to encourage because arm motion isn't involved. He also may be successful at tennis or golf because both sports require bent knees with straight arms. Over time, perhaps he will get better at other sports.

CRAWLING FOR ADULTS!

Adults with STNR problems can also improve their lives. Dr. O'Dell and Dr. Cook have witnessed over and over again that when children are tested and treated for the STNR problem, their parents realize that they have the problem, too. For example, a mother in her forties brought her son to see O'Dell and Cook. The mother worked diligently with her son, and he improved greatly. She had always wanted to play racquetball but was too uncoordinated. She was a very bright lady but had always had trouble doing more than one thing at a time. For example, she couldn't listen to music or the TV while she was trying to fix dinner. So her husband did the exercises with her. The result? She could fix dinner and listen to music at the same time. As a child she'd never been able to jump rope. After the exercises she was able to jump rope. Once she started, she didn't want to stop! She was further delighted to find that she could also play racquetball. So it's not the crawling in itself that's important. It's all the exciting activities that proper crawling can lead a person to do.

STUDIES OF STNR

Scientists have known for some time that the STNR is present in children at approximately six months until two years of age. In 1971, pioneer Miriam Bender, Ph.D., who had a background in physical therapy, studied the STNR in sixty-nine school children who were learning disabled and sixty children who were getting good grades in school. Seventy-five percent of the children with learning disabilities showed more signs of an immature STNR compared with the controls.[6]

Dr. Bender's graduate students, Nancy O'Dell and Patricia Cook continued her studies of STNR and are still extending their research and treatment of children with learning and/or behavior problems. In one study, Dr. O'Dell randomly placed sixty-nine children who had an immature STNR and learning difficulties in four different treatment groups. One group performed the exercises in Dr. Bender's program. Another group was given gross motor exercises. A third group performed perceptual exercises. The fourth group was not given any exercises and continued their regular classroom activities. This went on for ten weeks. Then tests were repeated. Those who had done the Bender exercises had matured their STNR. Their reading ability was significantly improved over that of the children in the regular classroom.[7]

Retired professors from the University of Indianapolis, Drs. O'Dell and

Cook continue their work at the Miriam Bender Diagnostic Center. They are currently studying fifty students in grades one through five at a school in a small town in Indiana. Teachers identified those children who showed characteristics of an immature STNR. Studies of the STNR status in these children were carried out, and behavior and learning tests were administered. Sixth-grade students, trained to administer STNR exercises, have been doing the crawling exercises with twenty-five children under the supervision of two teachers who are trained in administering these exercises. The other twenty-five students are not getting any exercises. At the end of the school year, they will repeat all the tests. The children will retake learning tests, and the teachers and parents will complete behavior questionnaires. More studies like this one need to be funded and the results evaluated so that skeptical teachers, psychologists, and physicians will recognize the importance of the status of the STNR in children with learning and behavior problems.

•

Crawling exercises are not a panacea for every child or adult. Some children and adults won't improve at all, while others will make remarkable improvements. But there are no adverse side effects, and the benefits last a lifetime.

WAY 12.
TRY BIOFEEDBACK

What is biofeedback? It is the use of sensors that record brain waves to monitor and ultimately control alertness. It is noninvasive and painless. The brain generates electricity. This electricity may be recorded by carefully "gluing" sensors on specific areas of the head. The biofeedback practitioner may also use caps containing the sensors that come in different sizes and are just pulled on over the head. The sensors send the electricity to an electroencephalograph (EEG), which transforms the electricity into patterns of waves. The EEG is similar to an electrocardiogram that records electrical impulses from the heart.

There are several kinds of waves with different heights and frequencies produced by the brain. With this technique, your child can use this feedback to see that his concentration is wavering and adjust it accordingly. Ultimately, the child learns to make these adjustments without the monitors. Delta waves are produced when your child sleeps. Theta waves are generated when your child relaxes. Alpha waves occur when your child is daydreaming. Sensorimotor rhythm (SMR) waves are the calm waves produced when the child is quietly alert with no fidgeting. Your child produces beta waves when he's thinking. You can see from these descriptions of the waves that your child will want to produce more of some waves and fewer of other waves, depending on the situation. In a learning situation, you would want your child to produce more beta waves and fewer alpha. It's not that some waves are bad. Your child needs them all. Biofeedback teaches him how to optimize the brain waves for better learning and behavior.

The EEG is connected to a computer that interprets the waves and transforms them into pictures on a screen. The pictures may be fish attempting to swim through a maze or someone playing basketball. If the child is concentrating, the fish successfully swim through the maze, but if the child is daydreaming, the action changes. If the child is not paying attention in the basketball game, his opponent scores. Alternatively, there may be a color display that lights up when appropriate brain waves are generated. There may be audio signals that tell your child how he is doing. Your child may receive points he can convert into small rewards. Biofeedback can improve attention, concentration, memory, eye-hand coordination, math skills, and problem solving.[1]

There are more than 300 facilities that are using biofeedback to treat ADHD. These include private clinics, university clinics, and schools with specially trained technicians. There are people with many different backgrounds trained in the use of biofeedback: pediatricians, psychiatrists, psychologists, teachers or counselors in special education, social workers, nurses, and other health-care providers.[2]

Improvement of symptoms vary from child to child but on the average, attention and concentration improve, organizational skills develop, and the child is less impulsive and hyperactive; so the child's behavior and learning skills improve, and he scores higher on intelligence tests. Handwriting may become more readable. Bed-wetting problems disappear. Speech difficulties, particularly articulation problems, may disappear. Social skills may improve. All of this leads to increased self-esteem.

Here's the case of ten-year-old John.[3] John was hyperactive and having trouble at school. Although he had an above average IQ, John was scheduled to repeat the fourth grade. His behavior at school disrupted the class, as John couldn't stay in his seat. John also showed a high degree of anxiety. Despite the use of Ritalin for a couple of years and placement in special education, John was still hyperactive and performing poorly in school. A psychologist found John to "exhibit motoric overactivity, extreme impulsivity, a short attention span, low frustration tolerance, high distractibility, and a rigid approach to the handling of his daily routine. In addition, his reading comprehension and word study skills were found to be lagging more than one year behind expected levels." John also had problems with proper eye movements.

Medication was stopped, and John started biofeedback. For the first three sessions, the biofeedback centered on helping John reduce muscle tension. Next, once a week for twenty sessions he received biofeedback to increase his SMR ("calm waves"). His hyperactivity improved dramatically. "His behavior was marked by the absence of overactivity, distractibility, and poor self-control. . . . He was noted to be, in all situations, more calm and under control than when he had been prescribed Ritalin."[4] His eye movements became normal and John began a program of reading remediation. Instead of being assigned to a special-education class, John was enrolled in a normal fourth-grade class. His grades were mostly As and Bs. Two years later, John had maintained all his improvements.

Perhaps you will identify with the problems of another child. Here's the story of Y.P., a thirteen-year-old who had been diagnosed as having ADHD by a psychiatrist.[5] The boy had been on and off Ritalin since first grade; the drug had provided only moderate help. Y.P. had also received individual counseling and group therapy. In school, he was disruptive and inattentive. He was in the sixth grade in special education classes for math, English, and spelling. He received below-average to average grades.

Baseline tests for Y.P. and behavioral questionnaires for his parents and teachers were administered prior to biofeedback. His brain waves were also monitored before and after. He completed thirty-five sessions in a three-month period using a system called Captain's Log. He liked the tasks and enjoyed earning rewards when he could alter his brain waves. At the end, the scores on his parents' questionnaire about his behavior had all improved. Some scores on the teachers' rating scale were higher and some were lower, but his teachers reported that he was more attentive and less disruptive in the classroom. His grades improved considerably—from Ds and Fs to Bs and Cs. His mother said that he was more attentive at home and could control his behavior. As the authors of this research report commented, "The most significant behavior change obtained with this child was the increase in on-task behaviors and reduction in disruptive behaviors at school."[6]

Then there was Donald, age thirteen, a very bright boy who just couldn't do his schoolwork, as it required him to listen to the whole problem or assignment. He constantly made careless errors. He was inattentive. Donald also had social problems. He alienated his peers and found it difficult to form lasting friendships. Adults considered him irritating and obnoxious. The researchers concluded: "When Donald increased his calm waves, it changed not only his approach to schoolwork but also his social interactions. He became considerate and polite and started making friends and building friendships."[7]

SCIENTIFIC STUDIES

In 1995, scientists reported a study of twenty-three children ages eight to nineteen.[8] They used both subjective and objective measures of changes before and after treatment. The researchers had developed a biofeedback technique to decrease excessive slow theta waves and to increase deficient beta waves when appropriate. Over the course of a summer, these children received intensive biofeedback training for one hour five days a week. The Test of Variables of Attention (TOVA) measured performance before and after all the biofeedback sessions. All the subjects improved on this objective computer test. Children on stimulant medication also improved on the TOVA, but the effects last only as long as the drug is in the bloodstream. Children receiving biofeedback are expected to maintain their improvements over time without more biofeedback.

The same scientists studied the effect of biofeedback on IQ scores. Subjects were chosen because IQ tests had been performed two years prior to the biofeedback, a length of time necessary because children generally improve on IQ tests if the tests are repeated within six months. Baseline EEG readings were taken at the beginning of the study. After forty biofeedback sessions over the course of a summer, all subjects in this study showed improved EEG findings and significantly higher IQ scores. The scientists concluded that on the basis of clinical experience, "it is clear that EEG biofeedback training for individuals with Attention Deficit Hyperactivity Disorder is a powerful adjunctive technique which is part of a multicomponent treatment process."[9]

In another 1995 study, scientists compared the effects of twenty sessions of biofeedback on symptoms of ADHD with results obtained with stimulant medication.[10] Forty-six patients, ages eight to twenty one, were chosen. The participants were divided into two groups of twenty-three subjects in each. One group received biofeedback, the other group received stimulant medication. The TOVA, an objective measure of attention and impulsivity, and speed of processing information, was administered to each subject before and after treatment. Teachers and parents completed behavior questionnaires. The group receiving biofeedback significantly improved their TOVA scores and the behavior measured. They showed improvements in attention, impulsivity, and processing speed. Parents and teachers reported better behavior and school performance. Next, the group who received biofeedback was compared with those who took medication. Both groups, those receiving the biofeedback and those receiving medication, experienced comparable improvements. The authors concluded: "The EEG biofeedback program is an effective treatment for AD/HD and may be the treatment of choice in cases where medication is ineffective, only partially effective, has unacceptable side effects, or where compliance with taking medication is low."[11]

ADVANTAGES AND DISADVANTAGES OF BIOFEEDBACK

Biofeedback has an advantage over medication in that there are no side effects. Furthermore, once improved, the child or adult will continue to maintain that improvement without the need for more biofeedback, so its effects are lifelong. However, biofeedback is expensive and time consuming. The initial screening may range from $300 to $700. Each session may cost between $60 and $120.[12] Usually a minimum of forty hour-long sessions are required. So parents must be willing and able to make the time and financial commitment.

•

Biofeedback is not a panacea for all children with ADD or ADHD. But it can be an important part of solving your child's hyperactivity puzzle.

PART 3

Helping Your Child Adjust to His New Diet

SHOPPING AND COOKING FOR YOUR ADD/ADHD CHILD

By now you should be able to determine what foods worsen your child's ADD/ADHD symptoms, and you must tailor his diet accordingly. But it seems like there is practically nothing left for him to eat. What are you to do? Don't be overwhelmed by the thought of shopping and cooking for your child with ADD/ADHD. Just take it one step at a time and do the best you can. It won't be long before shopping and cooking for your family become routine. In this chapter, I'll show you how to get started.

READING FOOD LABELS

Now that you know what foods and ingredients your child cannot eat, you'll have to become a careful label reader. You will need to know the ingredients in every food you give your child. You'll also want to know the nutritional value of these foods. First, look for the list of ingredients.

The ingredients are listed in descending order of the amount present in the product. For example, a package of rye crackers lists the ingredients whole rye, corn bran, salt, and caraway. So not surprisingly, rye is the greatest component and caraway the least. Notice, though, that these crackers unexpectedly contain corn, which could bother the corn-sensitive child. Here's another example: The ingredients on a bottle of barbecue sauce are listed as tomato puree (water, tomato paste), high fructose corn syrup, distilled vinegar, corn syrup, brown sugar, molasses, salt, cornstarch, natural flavors, spice, dehydrated onion, and mustard bran. Tomato puree appears to be the primary ingredient. Yet this barbecue sauce also contains sugar in four different forms—high fructose corn syrup, corn syrup, brown sugar, and molasses. The total sugars may exceed the amount of the tomato puree! So read ingredient lists carefully.

Also look for the "Nutrition Facts" on most labels. This label lists the amounts of each nutrient found in the food. The figure on page 173 is an example of the new food labels found on most foods. The serving size for this frozen dinner is 1 cup; there are about two and one half servings in a container. There are 500 calories in one serving, with 330 of them coming from fat. So 66 percent of the calories in this food comes from fat! That's a lot.

The percent (%) Daily Value is the amount of a day's nutrients found in one serving for someone consuming 2,000 calories a day. These Percent Daily Values include those for total fat, saturated fat, cholesterol, sodium, total carbohydrates, dietary fiber, and protein. Sugars, both added and naturally occurring, are listed in grams per serving. Four grams of sugar equal 1 teaspoon. This product contains 5 grams. One serving of this food provides no vitamin A or vitamin C but 20 percent of the calcium and 6 percent of the Daily Value for iron.

Don't be misled by products that proclaim in large print that they are "pure," "natural," "100 percent natural," or "all natural." Careful reading of the fine print on the labels may reveal artificial ingredients such as artificial colors, flavors, and preservatives. Further, there is often sugar in these products.

Start by reading labels of foods in your own cupboards that your family eats most often. Are they artificially colored and flavored? Such terms as "color added," "artificial color," "U.S. Certified Colors," "tartrazine," and "yellow dye #5" all mean that artificial color has been added. If the label says "naturally colored with carotene," the product may be okay. Carotene, saffron, turmeric, cochineal, and annatto are all natural dyes and not chemically related to the coal tar dyes. However, allergic reactions to cochineal and annatto have been reported. If a product is artificially flavored, the

Nutrition Facts

Serving Size 1 cup (249 gram)
Servings per Carton about 2½

Amount per Serving

Calories 500   Calories from Fat 330

	% Daily Value*
Total Fat 36g	56%
Saturated fat 22g	100%
Cholesterol 110mg	35%
Sodium 910mg	37%
Total Carbohydrate 33g	11%
Dietary Fiber 3g	13%
Sugars 5g	
Protein 12g	

Vitamin A 0% • Vitamin C 0% • Calcium 20% • Iron 6%

*Percent Daily Values are based on a 2,000 calorie diet. Your Daily Values may be higher or lower depending on your calorie needs:

Nutrient		2,000 Calories	2,500 Calories
Total Fat	Less than	65g	80g
Sat Fat	Less than	20g	25g
Cholestoral	Less than	300mg	300mg
Sodium	Less than	2,400mg	2,400mg
Total Carbohydrates		300g	375g
Fiber		25g	30g

Calories per gram:
Fat 9 • Carbohydrates 4 • Protein 4

Nutrition Facts Label

label should read "artificial flavoring." If it's artificial vanilla that's used, the label may say "vanillin." Citrus oils and cinnamon are natural flavors, but they may bother sensitive children.

Do the products in your cupboards contain preservatives? When shopping, look on the labels for such chemicals as BHA (butylated hydroxyanisole), BHT (butylated hydroxytoluene), sodium nitrite or nitrate, and sodium benzoate and avoid them.

Which products contain sugar? Staples like ketchup, table salt, mayonnaise, pickles, bread, jams, jellies, and many others all commonly contain sugar or corn sweeteners. You'll also need to know which products contain the natural foods you will be eliminating on the Common Foods Elimination Diet—milk, egg, corn, wheat, rye, chocolate, cola, sugar, legumes, and citrus. Later in this chapter, I'll give you tips for replacing these common foods in your child's diet.

It is hoped that the whole family will be living on the diet, so it's best not to have any of these products in the house. Get all of the foods not permitted out of your cupboards and refrigerator. Cravings for forbidden foods can be very strong and it's easier if these tempting foods aren't around.

GROCERY SHOPPING

Grocery shopping may become a little more complicated and time-consuming for you now. Plan to spend some time reading labels and getting ideas before and during your shopping trip. At first, beginning any new diet can be overwhelming, as can the necessary shopping. Ultimately, you will find shopping to be a breeze as you begin to automatically bypass the items you and your child must now avoid. Shop without your children if possible. Otherwise, shopping will take twice as long, and your concentration will be interrupted. After your child has been on his diet awhile and has lost his sugar craving and is more reasonable, you can take him shopping with you and help him to become a careful label reader. After all, someday he will be on his own, and shopping will be his responsibility. If he's used to treats when you go shopping, take along some carrots, nuts, crackers, fruit, or a healthy cookie (see recipes on pages 210–213).

Let's take an imaginary shopping trip. We'll go down each aisle, as they are set up in my supermarket. First we come to the packaged processed luncheon meats, bacon, and sausage. These may contain artificial colors and flavors, preservatives, sugar, corn, and milk. There will probably be nothing you can purchase from that array. You can easily make your own homemade sausage. Bypass the deli section of your store. Consult a cookbook or the directions that accompany a sausage maker for instructions. You will probably be able to find additive- and filler-free hot dogs and bologna at your health-food store. Hot dogs are near and dear to many children's hearts! Don't buy self-basting turkeys (they contain artificial coloring and butter), but you should be able to find frozen turkeys that haven't been processed or fresh turkeys, especially around Thanksgiving and Christmas. Read the labels on frozen fish. Try to find brands without additives. Don't buy breaded fish, which contains wheat, egg, sugar, and color. Better yet, visit the seafood department and choose fresh fish, especially the omega-3 fatty acid rich coldwater fish (fresh tuna, salmon, flounder, sardines, etc.). Choose fresh, lean meats and poultry in your meat department.

Our next aisle has candy on one side, pasta products on the other. Forget the candy and gum. Even some marshmallows have some dye in them, not to mention all the sugar they contain. You may want to buy your pasta products at your health-food store, where you can find them made from whole grains. For those sensitive to wheat, you can find pastas made from corn, rice, and spelt. DeBoles, Mrs. Leepers, and VitaSpelt are some brands to look for. As far as pasta sauces are concerned, almost all contain sugar or corn syrup. There are a few sauces that can be found in health-food stores that contain no additional sugar. Those made by Seeds of Change contain no sugars whatsoever. Read labels carefully. Make your own macaroni with real cheese. Buy only brown, unprocessed rice. Avoid rice mixes, which contain MSG, sugar, and corn.

Next come the canned meats, fish, and soups. Many brands of tuna and salmon are fine, but forget the hash, meat spreads, stews, etc. (They contain colors, nitrites, corn, and sugar.) Most soups, broths, and bouillon cubes contain sugar, MSG, corn sweeteners, and proteins, possibly partially hydrogenated oils, the preservative BHT, caramel coloring, soy protein, and wheat. You can shop at your health-food store for broth and soups. Or you can use the recipes for chicken and beef stocks in the recipes section (page 197) to easily make your own. On the other side of the aisle are crackers and cookies. If you look carefully, you may be able to find some whole-grain crackers such as RyKrisp or Wasa crackers that are free of sugar, colors, and preservatives. You may be able to find all-rice crackers or rice cakes at your grocery or health-food store.

As we go down the next aisle, there are such beverages as tea and cocoa. You may be able to find some herb teas that everyone can enjoy that do not contain caffeine. Don't buy cocoa or chocolate drinks; even the carob drink has sugar added. On the other side of this aisle are condiments. All ketchups contain sugar and/or corn sweeteners, though Westbrae makes a ketchup sweetened with only apple or pear juice concentrate. Some of them contain red dye to make them look redder than tomatoes. Some other ketchups at health-food stores contain honey. Barbecue sauces also contain sugar. See page 207 for a recipe for sugar-free barbecue sauce. Pickles will probably be out (they contain colors, sugar, and corn syrup), but you may be able to locate capers, which substitute well for chopped pickles. You should be able to find a brand of mustard that's okay. Look for a sugar- and egg-free mayonnaise at your health-food store. Nasoya is one such brand. Salad dressings generally contain sugar, artificial colors, egg, and corn. Newman's Own, Spectrum Naturals, Cardini's, and Annie's Naturals are some brands that make dressings that don't contain those ingredients. If you cannot find a suitable dressing, making your own is easy and economical. See page 206 for a recipe.

Now we come to the canned fruits and vegetables. Read labels carefully. Many canned vegetables contain artificial colors, corn sweeteners, and sugars. Some beans are dyed. Look for fruit packed in its own juice, not in syrup—light or heavy. Fruit cocktails usually have artificially colored maraschino cherries, not to mention extra sugar. You should be able to find sugar-free applesauce; Mott's Whole Foods and Leroux Creek make good versions. When choosing dried fruits, look for sun-dried fruits in your grocery and avoid those that contain sulfur dioxide. Many of the bottled fruit drinks and juices are a disaster (they contain artificial colors, sugar, and corn syrup). Choose only unsweetened 100 percent pure fruit juices such as orange, apple, pineapple, grape, grapefruit, and tomato.

As you know from reading about cereals in Part 1, many cereals are loaded with sugar, artificial colors, and preservatives. If your child isn't sensitive to grains, you might see what cereals your health-food store offers. Make sure you read all labels. Even some corn flakes found in health-food stores may contain added sugar. Barbara's, Health Valley, Arrowhead Mills, Kashi, Breadshop's, and Lifestream make cereals that contain no sugar or are sweetened with fruit juice. Instant breakfast drinks are out. You can easily make your own fruit smoothies. (See page 219.)

You must bypass all the cake mixes, prepared icings, pie crusts, gelatin mixes, puddings, and so on, for obvious reasons. Do look for unflavored gelatins. In the flour aisle, buy unbleached white or, better yet, stone-ground whole wheat, which is more nutritious, if your child is not sensitive to wheat. In the beginning of your new diet, while your family is still adjusting to change, you may want to mix whole wheat with unbleached flour so the texture won't be quite so coarse. Whole-wheat pastry flour is finer and works well in cookies, pancakes, and muffins. You may be able to find rye, oat, potato, rice, quinoa, and amaranth flours in your grocery, or you may have to go to the health-food store. Look for cold-pressed soy or canola oils at your grocery or health-food store.

Read the labels on any spices you buy. Most are fine but occasionally you'll find MSG, artificial colors, or dextrose added. Buy only pure extracts—vanilla, orange, lemon, lime, peppermint, and almond. Shredded coconut often has added sugar and artificial flavor, so you need to buy only unsweetened pure coconut, probably from a health-food store. Forget all the chocolate and look for some unsweetened carob powder. Be aware, though, that carob powder may contain cinnamon and citrus oils, though the label may be marked only as "natural flavoring." Choose only nuts that have no preservatives, oils, or sugar. Raw, unprocessed nuts are best. You'll have to locate some sugar-free salt and corn-free baking powder, probably at your health-food store.

Choose plenty of fresh vegetables and fruits, keeping in mind that you must avoid corn and citrus fruits on the Common Foods Elimination Diet and thereafter if your child is sensitive to them. Just a few words of caution: Vegetables such as zucchini, rutabagas, squash, cucumbers, and green peppers are often waxed and should be avoided or peeled, as the chemicals are not water-soluble and can't be washed away. Apples are also sometimes waxed. Choose dull, unwaxed-looking apples, or peel them before eating. Fruits and vegetables are also often treated with pesticides. Studies show that domestically grown apples, grapes, green beans, peaches, pears, spinach, and winter squash contain much higher levels of toxic chemicals than other foods studied. Common foods with low residues of pesticides include apple juice, bananas, broccoli, canned peaches, milk, orange juice, and canned or frozen corn and peas. Researchers think that pesticide residues pose more of a threat to the health of children than they do to adults. In children, they may adversely affect the developing central nervous system. Overall, organically grown produce is your best bet. It costs a little more, but it is certainly worth it.

This is a good time to choose fruits and vegetables you seldom eat, such as papayas, honeydew melons, sweet potatoes, squash, etc., as your child is much less likely to be sensitive to foods he's rarely eaten. In the produce area of my grocery store, there are jars of citrus fruits. Some contain sugar and others contain sodium benzoate, so it's best to section your own grapefruit and oranges rather than buying the jarred fruit, if your child can have citrus fruits. The fruit dips contain artificial colors and corn syrup, while the vegetable dips contain preservatives. Instead, make your own. (See page 205.)

Most foods from the dairy case will be off-limits during the Common Foods Elimination Diet (milk products, cheeses, and eggs). If your child is not sensitive to milk, use only low-fat white milk, not chocolate milk. For the Common Foods Elimination Diet, you should try to locate a margarine (butter is a milk product) with a safflower base that is naturally colored with carotene. Try your health-food store, but even there it's hard to find one that doesn't contain partially hydrogenated oils. Most margarines contain milk, corn oil, and coloring, either annatto or yellow #5 and #6. Another option is to clarify your butter; that is, remove the allergenic milk solids. Just melt your butter over low heat. Then set it aside for a few minutes to let the milk solids settle. Skim the butter fat from the top and then refrigerate. Discard the milk solids. If your child isn't sensitive to milk, there are a few brands of uncolored butter available. Manufacturers add coloring (usually annatto) to butter to standardize the yellow shade, as the color of butter varies with the time of year and whether the cows are grazing in the pastures or eating in the barn. Land O Lakes unsalted butter is never colored. The yellow cheeses are usually colored with annatto or carotene. When buying sour cream, whipping cream, cottage cheese, and yogurt, remember you are buying milk products and you should choose brands with the fewest additives. Gums are often added as stabilizers, and some people are sensitive to them. Choose only plain yogurt, as varieties with fruit unfortunately contain sugar or aspartame. You'll also find yeast cakes or dry yeast packages in the refrigerator case. Buy a brand without preservatives.

If your child is not sensitive to wheat, make sure you purchase whole-grain breads that list a whole grain as the first ingredient. Some breads contain caramel color to make them look healthier or more wholesome. Yellow dye may also be added to baked goods to make you think the product contains eggs. Most bread is made with bleached flour, lots of sugar, partially hydrogenated vegetable oils, and preservatives. Of course, there's the basic problem of wheat itself for some children. Oat, barley, and rye commercial breads always have wheat added. You may have to bake your own bread, rolls, and buns. You may decide to invest in a bread maker. Making baked goods without wheat and rye is not as simple as baking with wheat; substitutions are suggested later in this chapter beginning on page 182.

Most jams and jellies contain sugar or corn syrup. But there are some all-fruit preserves. Use them in small amounts because they contain concentrated natural sugars. Choose peanut butter made of only peanuts and salt. If you're avoiding peanuts on the Common Foods Elimination Diet, look for cashew or almond butter at your health-food store.

In the freezer case, choose unbuttered vegetables and nonsweetened fruits. For an occasional treat, you can find vanilla ice cream that is sweetened with aspartame. Some children do okay with small amounts of this on special occasions. Others are bothered by the milk and the aspartame. Most health-food stores carry Rice Dream Non-Dairy Dessert, which is milk- and sweetener-free. Most flavored ice pops are a disaster—they are full of sugar and artificial colors and flavors. Dole Fruit Juice Bars do not contain artificial colors or flavors, but they do contain sorbitol and aspartame. You can easily make your own flavored ices at home. Simply freeze some unsweetened juice with no artificial colors or flavors in an ice cube tray or ice pop containers. Read all labels on frozen fruit juices. Many contain sugar or corn syrup, and a few, like lime juice, contain dyes.

In the next aisle are snack foods on one side and soft drinks on the other. If your child can tolerate corn, Seyfert's low-fat baked tortilla chips and Bite-Size baked Tostitos, which contain just corn and salt, are good snack ideas. Tostitos all-natural salsa contains only a slight amount of sugar and is a good accompaniment to these chips. If your child can tolerate wheat, Mike-Sells sourdough nugget pretzels and Snyder's of Hanover sourdough hard pretzels are made of white flour, but they don't contain "bad" fats or sugar. Also, look for whole-wheat pretzels made with whole-wheat flour and no sugar or partially hydrogenated fats. Natural GH Foods makes a whole-wheat pretzel filled with peanut butter. Try to avoid the baked potato chips found in grocery stores, as they all seem to contain bad fats and sugar. Look for potato chips baked with no sugar or bad fats. Terra Chips makes different exotic-colored vegetable chips, including yucca, sweet potato, and taro, cooked in canola oil. They are lower in total and saturated fat than regular potato chips.

On the opposite side of this row are the soft drinks. Buy some club soda and add it to fruit juice to make your own version of soda. Later on, when your child is doing well, you might try a few ounces of uncolored diet soft drinks such as 7Up, Sprite, and Squirt on special occasions. These contain citrus extracts and aspartame.

•

As you can see, much of your shopping may now need to be done at a health-food store, where you can more readily find products without additives that your child cannot tolerate. Some health-food stores carry items containing artificial colors and flavors, preservatives, and lots of sugar, which may be labeled "raw sugar," "brown sugar," "cane sugar," or "turbinado sugar." Watch out for these products and avoid them. You'll soon find that your grocery shopping goes quickly. You'll automatically pass by many areas and know exactly what brands you're looking for. It's not a bad idea to keep reading labels from time to time, even on those products that you find do not have intolerable additives, as manufacturers change their products over time.

COOKING WITHOUT THOSE COMMON FOODS THAT MAY TRIGGER REACTIONS

By now you may be wondering, "How am I ever going to avoid these foods and feed my family appealing, nutritious meals?" Here are suggestions for some substitutions.

Milk

There are lots of substitutions for milk, but you'll soon get a knack for determining which one will taste best in a given recipe. Also, you will want to read the label to see how much calcium your child will be getting. (One cup of cow's milk has about 300 milligrams of calcium and 100 international units of vitamin D.) Try Enriched Rice Dream Milk from your grocery or health-food store. It's made from a rice base, is not sweetened, and is fortified with calcium and vitamin D. Soymilk is another good alternative. Some brands are fortified with calcium and vitamin D. Both Rice Dream and soymilk can be substituted cup for cup for cow's milk. You can make your own banana "milk" at home. It works well for cereals. Combine one-half small banana and 1 cup water in a blender. Blend on the highest speed until smooth. Use immediately. Nut "milk" also works well for cereals. Combine one-third cup unprocessed walnuts, sliced almonds, sliced pecans, or sunflower seeds with 1 cup water in a blender. Blend on the highest speed until smooth. Nut milk tastes best fresh, but you can refrigerate the leftovers. It can be used up to one to two days after making.

Substitute unsweetened pineapple juice for milk measure for measure in recipes that call for milk. This works surprisingly well in waffles, pancakes, muffins, or biscuits. Use chicken stock to substitute for milk cup for cup in cream soups and casseroles. For example, you can make "creamy" tomato soup using chicken stock, tomato paste, and seasonings. Chicken stock also works well in fish chowder. You might want to thicken the stock with some cornstarch or arrowroot powder first for a nice creamy consistency. When making mashed potatoes, you can use a little of the water left over from boiling the potatoes instead of milk; or use Enriched Rice Dream Milk.

Eggs

Eggs act as leavening agents in recipes, making the finished product lighter. Eggs also bind ingredients together, keeping the finished product from crumbling. So cooking without eggs is difficult in some types of recipes, but generally you should be able to get around using eggs in a recipe. Cookies and quick breads often turn out well without eggs. If you have a recipe for one of these that calls for eggs, try omitting the eggs. When making egg-free cookies, grease and lightly flour the cookie sheet to prevent the cookies from spreading. You may be tempted to use an egg substitute in recipes, but be careful: despite the term, egg substitutes, such as Egg Beaters, usually contain egg whites. Try an egg-free commercial substitute such as Jolly Joan Egg Replacer. Follow the directions on the package. Use the recipe for Apricot Egg Replacer on page 213 to replace eggs in meatloaf, muffins, and quick breads. In muffins, pancakes, and quick breads, substitute for 1 egg: 2 tablespoons of allowed starch flour, one-half tablespoon of allowed butter or margarine, one-half teaspoon baking powder, and 2 tablespoons of liquid.

Corn, Wheat, and Rye

There are several alternatives you can use for wheat, but don't be surprised if they don't have the taste and texture you get with wheat. Rye and barley flours are similar to wheat, but most children who are sensitive to wheat are also sensitive to rye and barley. There are also several alternatives to the use of cornstarch in recipes.

For thickening, 1 tablespoon cornstarch equals any one of the following:

- 1 tablespoon arrowroot
- 2 tablespoons wheat flour

- 1 tablespoon potato starch flour
- 1 tablespoon rice flour
- 4 teaspoons quick-cooking tapioca

For 1 cup wheat flour substitute one of the following:

- 1 cup amaranth
- 1 cup quinoa
- ½ cup arrowroot
- ½ cup barley flour
- ¾ cup buckwheat flour
- 1 cup corn flour
- 1⅓ cups finely ground oats or oat flour
- ⅝ cup potato starch or potato flour
- ¾ to ⅞ cup rice flour
- 1⅓ cups soy flour
- 1 cup tapioca flour

Sometimes it works better to substitute a combination of flours for 1 cup wheat flour:

- ⅝ cup rice flour plus ⅓ cup potato flour
- ⅝ cup rice flour plus ⅓ cup rye flour
- 1 cup soy flour plus ¼ cup potato starch
- ½ cup cornstarch plus ½ cup potato flour

For thickening, 1 tablespoon wheat flour equals any one of these:

- 1½ teaspoons cornstarch
- 1½ teaspoons arrowroot
- 1½ teaspoons potato starch
- 1½ teaspoons rice flour
- 2 teaspoons quick-cooking tapioca

Instead of spaghetti and noodles, try Chinese bean threads, rice, rice flour noodles, spaghetti squash, corn pasta, and rice vermicelli.

Chocolate

Carob is a healthy, delicious, easy, and naturally sweet substitute for chocolate. Replace cocoa with carob powder measure for measure. Replace 1 square of unsweetened chocolate with 3 tablespoons carob powder, plus 1 extra tablespoon vegetable oil or butter. Replace chocolate chips with finely chopped dried fruits such as apricots, figs, and especially dates in appropriate recipes for a tasty, healthier alternative.

Sugar

Your child may be following a low- or no-sugar diet. In many recipes, you can simply omit the sugar. For example, some recipes for spaghetti sauce call for sugar. Just leave it out. Likewise, many commercial brands of spaghetti sauce contain sugar or corn sweeteners. Who needs sweet-tasting spaghetti sauce? If you make your own bread, you most likely add some sugar to help the yeast multiply so that the bread rises. Just leave it out. Your bread will rise just fine without sugar, although it may take a little longer. In recipes for muffins, waffles, or biscuits omit the sugar. Top with a dab of all-fruit preserves or Blueberry Syrup (see page 203) or Strawberry Sauce (see page 204). Or choose a recipe that calls for sweet-tasting fruit, such as apples, pears, or blueberries. Replace milk with unsweetened pineapple juice to add extra sweetness. You can even make ice cream without any artificial sweeteners. Just add concentrated orange juice or unsweetened pineapple juice to sweeten the ice cream. Adding raisins or chopped dates to recipes will sweeten foods without any added table sugar or artificial sweeteners. If your child tolerates artificial sweeteners, use them sparingly. One packet of sweetener is equal to 2 teaspoons of sugar.

•

Cooking without some of your favorite foods will be a challenge, but by choosing alternative ingredients and modifying your recipes, you can stick to your child's diet but still eat well.

CELEBRATING
HAPPY HOLIDAYS

If your child has behavior problems, they probably are exaggerated at holiday and party times. Anticipation and excitement coupled with eating foods that are high in sugars, artificial ingredients, and foods to which your child is sensitive lead to tears, tantrums, and a trying time for all.

There are three ways to handle holidays and parties. The first way is to just "blow the diet" and let your child eat what he wants with the explicit understanding that the diet will resume as soon as the holiday is over. The disadvantage of this approach is that your child may be out of control and ruin the holiday for everyone. The second way is to limit the amounts of forbidden foods. Talk with your child before the holiday and settle on how much of each food or candy he can have—perhaps one small slice of cake or three pieces of candy. Emphasize the foods that he enjoys and can safely eat. The third way is to stick to the diet but provide alternative treats. Talk with your child about the coming holiday or party and explain that he won't be able to eat some things that he has eaten in the past. List the foods that he can have, especially the ones he likes best. If he understands the situation, you have a good chance of getting his cooperation. You'll have to choose which approach works best for your family.

Providing special food for holidays and birthdays while taking care of diet needs may seem to be an impossible task. For some holidays, such as Halloween and Easter, candy and sweets are, unfortunately, a main attraction, especially for children. Some rethinking must be done to come up with ideas that still lend a festive holiday feeling but are nutritious and follow dietary needs of family members.

First, a positive attitude is imperative. If you are the cook in the family, you must be determined to serve attractive, nutritious meals and snacks that everyone can eat. Do this cheerfully so others in the family will come to meals in the right frame of mind. This is especially important at the beginning of the diet. The stakes are high for your child, making all the extra effort well worth your time and energy.

Second, don't feel that you must serve a wide variety of foods. A simple, carefully prepared menu is far better than making a lot of dishes that leave you harried and frustrated. Select the things in the diet that your family enjoys the most and take special care when shopping to buy the best quality meats, fruits, and vegetables you can afford. Add garnishes such as parsley or fruit slices to platters of meats or casseroles to make a pleasing appearance.

Plan menus ahead and do as much preparation as possible beforehand. Ask for helpers in the kitchen. Even small children can do things to help and this gives them a good feeling about themselves.

Don't abandon all your old recipes. If you review holiday menus you have used in the past, you will probably find that many recipes are fine to use as they are. Even if they have forbidden ingredients, don't be afraid to try substitutions. Try an egg replacer in baked items. Substitute oat, rice, amaranth, or quinoa flours for wheat flour. Milk can be omitted by substituting water, or fruit juice if flavoring and sweetness are desired. Or try Enriched Rice Dream Milk or soymilk.

Fifth, when invited to friends' houses for holidays, offer to bring a dish your child likes and can eat. Perhaps the hostess will understand your problem and provide some alternative foods for your child that everyone will enjoy.

Here are some suggestions for individual holidays. You'll have to adapt the menus and recipes to your child's own diet.

THANKSGIVING

At Thanksgiving, a turkey dinner is a must at our house. A typical menu might be:

- Roast Turkey with Bread Stuffing (see page 199)
- Cranberry sauce
- Mashed potatoes with homemade gravy
- Mashed sweet potatoes
- Frozen peas
- Wheat Bread (see page 214) or Rice Muffins (see page 196)
- Pumpkin Pie (see page 214)

Choose a fresh turkey that is not self-basting. Stuff it with bread stuffing using whole-wheat bread. If your child is sensitive to wheat, try a rice stuffing instead. Thicken gravy with cornstarch, tapioca, or potato starch as suggested on pages 182–183. Commercial cranberry sauce is full of corn sweeteners, but making your own is a snap. Just boil the cranberries in water until they pop. Stir in thawed concentrated unsweetened frozen 100 percent fruit juice, artificial sweetener, or stevia to taste, and chill. Mash either potatoes or sweet potatoes with Rice Dream Milk or soymilk. Don't use instant mashed potatoes, packaged stuffings, or prepared gravies, as they are usually full of additives, artificial colors, preservatives, milk, or other problem foods.

CHRISTMAS

Christmas should also be a special celebration. For Christmas parties, try the Pumpkin Cookies (page 210), Vanilla Cookies (page 211), Oatmeal Cookies (page 212), Cinnamon Cookies (page 210), and Thumbprint

Cookies (page 213). Put out bowls of unprocessed nuts. (If you like roasted nuts better, just toss them with a little soy or canola oil and toast them on a cookie sheet in the oven until they are slightly brown. Lightly salt.) Serve a platter of fresh veggies or colorful fruits with dips. The drinks can be simple—unsweetened 100 percent pure fruit juice over ice served with holiday cups and napkins. Unsweetened cherry-cranberry juice is colorful and delicious. These things can be enjoyed, and they keep your child on his diet without his even realizing it.

Christmas dinner could be prepared using the following menu:

- Pot roast with gravy
- Scalloped potatoes
- Baked acorn squash
- Tossed salad with Italian Dressing (see page 206)
- Wheat rolls
- Apple Cake (see page 207) with Whipped Topping (page 204)

If wheat is a problem, thicken the gravy with alternative thickeners found on pages 182–183. The squash can be served with just a little butter or allowed margarine. Instead of making Wheat Bread (page 214), use the same dough to make rolls. Even though the menu is varied, you have a hearty holiday meal for family and guests that can be handled relatively easily.

Skip the candy cane and other sweet treats in stuffing the stocking. Instead, include an orange and some small toys—small cars, card games, a yo-yo, a stuffed animal, crayons, special pencils and pens, and so on.

NEW YEAR'S DAY

An open house for friends and neighbors can be a great way to start the new year. Include the children as well as the adults. Make your own cheese balls with real cheese. Serve nuts, allowed pretzels and chips, or popcorn. A raw vegetable tray with dip will be appreciated by many who are trying to keep their calories down. Serve hot apple juice simmered with cinnamon sticks. The aroma will fill your house with holiday cheer. Choose items your child can eat so he feels that he and other children are a part of the party, even though everything is nutritious and adheres to his diet.

EASTER

Easter is another holiday that seems to revolve around candy and sweets. Skip the candy in the Easter basket. Instead include small age-appropriate toys. If you want to dye eggs, your child can have fun using natural dyes. Here are some easy ideas: To dye eggs blue, add 1 tablespoon vinegar to 1 cup blueberry or grape juice. Eggs turn a pretty bluish-lavender color. To dye eggs brown, add 2 tablespoons vinegar to a cup of coffee. To dye eggs pink, add 2 tablespoons vinegar to 1 cup beet juice. To dye eggs yellow, add 1 teaspoon saffron to 1 cup water and boil slowly for about 5 minutes. Cool and strain. Add 1 tablespoon vinegar to 1 cup of the saffron dye and submerge egg. This dye will color eggs bright yellow.

For Easter dinner serve:

- Roast leg of lamb with gravy
- Au gratin potatoes
- Cooked carrots
- Wheat Bread (see page 214)
- Orange Ice Cream (see page 217) or Rice Dream Non-Dairy Dessert (found in most health-food stores)

Roast the leg of lamb and reserve the drippings to make your own gravy. Skip the mint jelly because of the artificial green dyes and sugar. Make your own au gratin potatoes using uncolored cheese or cheese colored with annatto. Orange Ice Cream is a nice finale to this holiday dinner. You can make it with frozen pineapple juice instead of orange juice.

FOURTH OF JULY

Fourth of July is an ideal time for a picnic. For the menu serve:

- Grilled hamburgers or allowed hot dog on buns
- Relish tray with Vegetable Dip (see page 205)
- Fruit Juice Gelatin (see page 216)
- Potato salad
- Watermelon fruit basket
- Cookies (see recipe section for several delicious recipes)

Look for frozen hot dogs at your health-food store. You may have to make your own buns. Just use the Wheat Bread recipe (see page 214) and divide into bun-sized portions. Let it rise, and bake. Grape juice with added fruit chunks makes a pretty looking substitute for commercial gelatins. Use your favorite potato salad recipe with allowed mayonnaise. To make the watermelon basket, cut a whole watermelon in half lengthwise. Scoop out the pulp, remove the seeds, and cut into 1-inch chunks. Cup up a variety of other fruits, such as honeydew melon, strawberries, raspberries, cantaloupe, grapes, kiwis, and pineapple. Just before the picnic, fill the melon half with the fruit by adding small amounts of each fruit until filled. Chill and serve with cookies.

HALLOWEEN

Candy is the main attraction at Halloween. Instead of handing out the usual "junk food" at trick-or-treat time, give apples, small boxes of raisins, special pencils, coins, and stickers.

Of course, your child will want to go trick-or-treating. Make it clear again that he will not be able to eat most of what he gets, and make sure you have treats on hand that are allowed. Maybe he would like to trade in his treats for a penny apiece. Or maybe you can establish a "Good Witch" holiday. The child chooses a couple of pieces of candy to eat on Halloween and the rest is left for the "Good Witch," who comes late at night and leaves a nice present. You can either pitch all the candy or take it to work for your coworkers.

You also might have a Halloween party for your child. The menu could include:

- Apple Cake (see page 207) with Whipped Topping (page 204), decorated as a pumpkin face
- Popcorn, nuts, or toasted seeds
- Hot apple cider
- Witches'-brew punch (see below)

Have the guests come in costume. Decorate the room with black and orange streamers and balloons. Paper skeletons and witches, ghosts made from old sheets, Indian corn and corn stalks will complete the decorations. Create a pumpkin centerpiece by carving a jack-o'-lantern and placing a candle inside. Activities can include bobbing for apples, pin the nose on the pumpkin, a treasure hunt, and ghost stories.

Serve all the food buffet-style and let everyone help himself. The pumpkin face cake is Apple Cake (page 207) "iced" with Whipped Topping (page 204) that has been colored with carrot juice. Make the face by outlining the eyes, nose, and mouth with raisins or nuts. The witches'-brew punch is a combination of favorite 100 percent fruit juices. Drop small pieces of dry ice into the punch to make it bubble and smoke.

BIRTHDAYS

Children always look forward to their birthdays with much excitement. This sometimes leads to behavior problems that make these occasions times of frustration and anxiety for the rest of the family.

For a very small child, a simple family party would be best. If you wish, invite one or two of your child's friends to join in the celebration with a treat of allowed ice cream and cake. As your child gets older and a party with several children seems more in order, try to build it around a special interest. Take some friends from the ball team to a local ball game with allowed ice cream and cake afterward. A luncheon party followed by a trip to the movies could be just right for your youngster.

Of course, the traditional type of birthday party with ice cream, games, and favors will always be a hit. Choose food that everyone will enjoy. Make your own Orange Ice Cream (see page 217; you could enlist everyone's help in turning the crank to make it), or buy Rice Dream Non-Dairy Dessert. Don't mention that the ice cream may be different from what kids normally eat—just serve it with a smile. Apple Cake (page 207) with Whipped Topping (page 204) works well as a birthday cake. If your child is sensitive to wheat, try making the cake with rice flour.

•

With a little planning, you can turn all your special family occasions into memorable, happy celebrations.

PLEASING RECIPES
FOR THE CHILD
WITH ADD/ADHD

These are some of the recipes my family has enjoyed over the years. They illustrate some of the easy ways you can still enjoy favorite foods without compromising nutrition or diet restrictions. Experiment with your own family's recipes. Try substituting or partially substituting whole-wheat or whole-wheat pastry flour for unbleached white flour. Replace bad fats with good fats. Use sweet fruits or concentrated fruit juices instead of sugar in appropriate recipes. Keep artificial sweeteners to a minimum.

BREAKFAST TREATS

• Cinnamon Toast •

This toast not only makes a tasty breakfast dish, it makes a delightful treat for any time of the day.   *Yield: 1 serving*

1 slice whole-grain bread
1 teaspoon butter or allowed margarine
Dash of cinnamon
½ packet Equal, Natra Taste, Sweet One, or Sweet'n Low

Toast bread lightly. Spread with butter. Sprinkle cinnamon on top. Place under broiler until butter melts. Remove from broiler. Sprinkle with sweetener. Serve immediately.

• French Toast •

Your child does not have to give up French toast. Just make it with whole-grain breads. If he is sensitive to milk, leave it out. Serve with Blueberry syrup or Strawberry Sauce. (See pages 203 and 204.)

Yield: 4 servings

2 eggs
2 tablespoons milk (optional)
⅛ teaspoon pure vanilla extract
4 slices whole grain bread

Beat together eggs, milk, and vanilla. Dip bread in egg mixture and fry in nonstick skillet. Serve with whipped light butter and fresh sliced fruits, Strawberry Sauce, or Blueberry Syrup.

• Pancakes •

Just because your child may be sensitive to several foods, you don't have to give up pancakes—just alter the ingredients. Leave out the sugar. Replace the "bad" fats with "good" fats. If your child is sensitive to milk, replace with water or pineapple juice. If your child is sensitive to eggs, replace with extra water and baking powder. And trade in the maple syrup for fruit, all-fruit jams, Strawberry Sauce (see page 203), or Blueberry Syrup (see page 204).   *Yield: 6 medium pancakes*

1¼ cups whole-wheat pastry flour

3 teaspoons baking powder

½ teaspoon salt

1 egg, beaten, or 2 tablespoons water and ½ teaspoon baking powder

1 cup plus 2 tablespoons milk, unsweetened pineapple juice, or water

2 tablespoons pure canola or soy oil

Stir dry ingredients together. Stir liquid ingredients together and add to dry ingredients. Stir until just mixed. Batter may be thinned as needed with extra milk, water, or juice. Bake on a nonstick grill or skillet. Serve hot with a small amount of whipped butter, sliced fresh fruits, small amounts of all-fruit jams, Strawberry Sauce, or Blueberry Syrup.

• Blueberry Muffins •

Serve these muffins for breakfast along with a good source of protein such as eggs, a cold chicken leg, a slice of cold roast beef, or yogurt.

Yield: 12 muffins

2 cups whole-wheat pastry flour

1½ teaspoons baking powder

1 teaspoon salt

1 egg, beaten

¾ cup milk or Enriched Rice Dream Milk

2 tablespoons pure canola, soy, or walnut oil

¼ cup concentrated frozen unsweetened white grape juice
or orange juice, thawed

1 cup fresh or frozen (thawed and drained) blueberries

In a large bowl, combine dry ingredients. In a separate bowl, stir together the remaining ingredients. Add the wet ingredients to the dry. Stir until just mixed. (The batter should be lumpy.) Oil a muffin tin and fill the cups two-thirds full. Bake at 400°F for 20 minutes. Serve warm.

• Rice Muffins •

In this easy muffin recipe, rice flour replaces wheat flour, apricot puree replaces egg, and water or fruit juice substitutes for milk.   *Yield: 12 muffins*

1½ cups rice flour

½ teaspoon salt

2 teaspoons baking powder

¼ teaspoon baking soda

4 tablespoons canola oil

3 tablespoons Apricot Egg Replacer (see page 213)

1 cup water or 100 percent pure fruit juice

Place all ingredients in a mixing bowl and stir until batter is smooth. Spoon batter into oiled muffin tin and bake at 350°F for 15 to 20 minutes.

• Sausage Patties •

Commercial sausage contains sweeteners, MSG, and nitrites; but it's easy to make your own. These patties are a tasty way to add protein to your breakfast.   *Yield: 12 patties*

2 pounds coarsely ground lean pork, beef, or turkey
4 teaspoons sage
1/2 teaspoon thyme
1/2 teaspoon marjoram
1/2 teaspoon basil
1 1/2 teaspoons black pepper
2/3 cup water

Combine all ingredients in a large mixing bowl. Mix thoroughly. Shape into twelve patties. Fry in nonstick skillet until fully cooked and slightly browned. Or package for freezing and use patties as needed.

SOUPS AND STOCKS

• Beef Stock •

Commercial canned beef stock contains MSG, caramel coloring, and sugar, and beef bouillon cubes contain all that plus partially hydrogenated fats. This recipe avoids all those problems and provides a nutritious base for soups.   *Yield: 1 1/2 quarts*

6 pounds beef soup bones
2 1/2 quarts cold water
1 medium onion, sliced, or 1/4 cup instant minced onion
1/2 cup chopped celery
1 bay leaf
Several sprigs fresh parsley, or 1 tablespoon dried flakes
Salt and pepper to taste

In a large pot or Dutch oven, cover beef bones with cold water. Bring to a boil, add onion, celery, bay leaf, and parsley. Bring slowly to a boil.

Reduce heat and simmer for 2 to 3 hours. Strain, season, and cool. Refrigerate. Skim off layer of fat from top when ready to use stock.

• Chicken Stock •

Commercial chicken stock contains MSG, sugar, and corn protein. Chicken bouillon cubes also contain sugar and MSG, plus partially hydrogenated oils and the preservative BHT. But it's easy to make your own. And I think this one tastes even better than the store-bought variety.

Yield: 2 quarts

4 pounds chicken bones or whole chicken, broken up
4 quarts cold water
1 medium onion, diced, or ¼ cup instant minced onion
1 carrot, diced
Several stalks celery, diced
Salt and pepper to taste

Cover chicken bones with cold water in a Dutch oven. Add onion, carrot, and celery and bring to a boil. Simmer, uncovered, for 2 to 3 hours. Strain, season, and cool. Refrigerate. Skim off layer of fat on top when ready to use stock.

• Chicken and Rice Soup •

Commercial chicken soup contains MSG. This recipe provides protein and whole-grain brown rice, without the MSG.   *Yield: 6 servings*

6 cups Chicken Stock (see recipe above)
½ cup uncooked brown rice
⅓ cup diced onion

¹/₃ cup diced celery

1 tablespoon olive oil

1 cup diced cooked chicken

2 tablespoons chopped fresh parsley

Salt

Heat chicken stock to boiling. Add rice. Cover and simmer 35 minutes. Sauté onion and celery in olive oil for about 5 minutes and add to soup. Add chicken, parsley, and salt to taste.

ENTRÉES AND SIDE DISHES

• Bread Stuffing •

This stuffing is nutritious and tasty. The bread is whole-grain, the applesauce adds a slightly sweet taste, and the oil contains omega-3 fatty acids.   *Yield: Stuffing for 10-pound turkey or chicken*

1¹/₂ teaspoons poultry seasoning (use a brand
   with no MSG)

¹/₄ teaspoon nutmeg

2 teaspoons salt

8 cups cubed whole-wheat bread

2 tablespoons grated onion

2 eggs, slightly beaten, or ¹/₂ cup unsweetened applesauce

¹/₂ cup pure canola or soy oil

Combine dry ingredients with bread cubes. Add onion, eggs, and oil. Mix well.

• Three-Bean Salad •

This colorful salad is delicious, nutritious, and easy to prepare. Kidney and navy beans are excellent sources of omega-3 fatty acids.

Yield: 6 to 8 servings

1 15-ounce can kidney beans, rinsed and drained

1 16-ounce can navy beans, rinsed and drained

1 16-ounce can green beans, rinsed and drained

¼ cup pure canola, soy, or walnut oil

⅔ cup vinegar

½ cup concentrated frozen apple juice, thawed

1 tablespoon minced dried onion, or ¼ cup chopped fresh onion

½ teaspoon salt

Mix together all ingredients. Chill overnight. Drain before serving.

• Chili •

This recipe is easy, inexpensive, and nutritious. The kidney beans, oil, and flaxseed are rich sources of essential omega-3 fatty acids.

Yield: 6 to 8 servings

1 pound lean ground meat

1 19-ounce can kidney beans, drained, ⅔ cup liquid reserved

1 15-ounce can tomato puree

1 tablespoon instant minced onion

2 tablespoons chili powder

2 tablespoons pure soy or canola oil

¼ cup ground flaxseed

Lightly brown meat in a hot nonstick pan. Drain off fat. Stir in remaining ingredients. Bring to a boil. Reduce heat, cover, and simmer 10 minutes.

• Meat Loaf •

This meat loaf is great for dinner or served cold for breakfast or lunch. It works well for the child who is sensitive to eggs or wheat.

Yield: 6 to 8 servings

2 pounds ground lean meat
1/3 cup minute tapioca
1/4 cup Apricot Egg Replacer (see recipe on page 213)
1/3 cup finely chopped onion, or
  1 tablespoon instant minced onion
1 1/2 teaspoons salt
1/4 teaspoon ground pepper
1 1/2 cups mashed canned tomatoes

Combine all ingredients, mixing well. Then pack into a 9×5-inch loaf pan. Bake at 350°F for 1 to 1¼ hours. Place loaf on serving platter and slice. May be served hot or cold.

• Pork Chops •

Apple juice adds delicious flavor and sweetness to meats and poultry. These pork chops can easily be reheated in the morning to provide protein for the start of a good day.

Yield: 4 servings

4 pork chops, cut 1-inch thick
1/4 cup water
1/2 cup concentrated frozen apple juice, thawed

Brown pork chops in a nonstick skillet. Place chops in an ovenproof dish. Add water. Season with salt and pepper. Spread concentrated apple juice on top of the chops. Cover and bake for 1 hour.

• Wheat-Free Spaghetti •

Some children with ADHD are sensitive to wheat, a hard ingredient to avoid. Try this delicious alternative to spaghetti. Spaghetti sauce (see below for recipe) can also be served over rice or rice noodles from a specialty foods store.   *Yield: 4 servings*

1 3½-to-4-pound spaghetti squash
2 cups allowed Spaghetti Sauce (see below)
Parmesan cheese (optional)

Cut squash in half lengthwise and scoop out seeds. Place halves face-down in a shallow dish and add about ½ inch water. Bake in oven at 350°F for 45 minutes to 1 hour, or until soft when pricked with a fork. Remove from oven. Drain thoroughly. Scoop squash from shell by running the tines of a fork lengthwise down the squash pulp so that it comes out in spaghetti-like strings. Top with sauce and Parmesan cheese.

• Spaghetti Sauce •

Commercial spaghetti sauce usually contains corn syrup or sugar. This recipe is tasty and nutritious. The meat provides protein and other nutrients; the tomatoes provide sweet flavor and nutrition; and the flaxseed adds good omega-3 fatty acids.   *Yield: 8 cups*

1½ pounds lean ground beef, pork, or turkey
3 cloves garlic
1 large onion, minced
1 28-ounce can whole tomatoes, undrained and slightly chopped
2 6-ounce cans tomato paste
1½ teaspoons oregano
1 teaspoon dried sweet basil
½ teaspoon thyme

1 bay leaf
1 teaspoon salt
¼ teaspoon pepper
1 cup water
¼ cup ground flaxseed

Brown the ground meat in a large nonstick skillet. Add garlic and onion and cook slightly. Add all other ingredients and bring to a boil. Cover, reduce heat, and simmer for approximately 1 hour. Add more water if necessary. Stir in flaxseed. Use immediately or store in freezer for future use.

SAUCES, DIPS, DRESSINGS, AND TOPPINGS

• Blueberry Syrup •

Serve this tasty topping over homemade pancakes, waffles, or French toast. Choose the sweetener your child tolerates best.   *Yield: 1½ cups*

1 12-ounce package frozen unsweetened blueberries, thawed
½ cup water
1 tablespoon butter or allowed margarine
¼ teaspoon nutmeg
1 tablespoon pure lemon juice
4 teaspoons cornstarch
¼ cup concentrated frozen unsweetened apple or white grape juice, thawed;
    6 packets Equal, Natra Taste, Sweet One, or Sweet'n Low; or a pinch
    of stevia

In a saucepan, combine blueberries with ⅜ cup water, butter or margarine, nutmeg, and lemon juice. Bring to a boil. Reduce heat and simmer until berries are soft. Dissolve cornstarch in remaining water. Add to blue-berry syrup and continue to cook, stirring constantly, until syrup thickens. Remove from heat and cool slightly. Stir in thawed juice or other sweet-ener. Serve warm or chilled.

• Strawberry Sauce •

Use this tasty, nutritious sauce instead of maple syrup for pancakes, waffles, or French toast.   *Yield: 2 cups*

2 cups frozen unsweetened strawberries, thawed
3 tablespoons water
2 teaspoons cornstarch
¼ teaspoon almond extract
¼ cup concentrated frozen unsweetened apple or white grape juice, thawed;
  6 packets Equal, Natra Taste, Sweet One, or Sweet'n Low; or a pinch
  of stevia

In a heavy saucepan, cook strawberries and 2 tablespoons of the water over medium heat until strawberries are soft. Dissolve cornstarch in the remaining 1 tablespoon cold water. Add to strawberries and cook, stirring constantly, until sauce thickens. Stir in almond extract. Remove from heat. Stir in fruit juice or other sweetener. Serve warm or chilled.

• Whipped Topping •

This topping makes a delicious icing for cakes. Because it is relatively high in saturated fats, though, use it sparingly.   *Yield: 1½ cups*

1 cup whipping cream
1 teaspoon pure vanilla extract

¹/₄ cup frozen concentrated unsweetened white grape, orange, or pineapple juice; 2 packets Equal, Natra Taste, Sweet One, or Sweet'n Low; or a pinch of stevia

Using an electric mixer, whip cream in a chilled bowl. Beat in vanilla and fruit juice or other sweetener. Serve immediately. Refrigerate leftover topping.

• Fruit Dip •

This tasty fruit dip will encourage your child to eat more fruits.

Yield: 1 cup

1 8-ounce carton plain yogurt
2 tablespoons all-fruit preserves
¹/₄ teaspoon cinnamon
1 teaspoon grated lemon rind (optional)

Combine ingredients, chill, and serve with fruit chunks.

• Vegetable Dip •

A tasty dip will help your child eat his veggies. Serve with an attractive array of carrots, cherry tomatoes, or broccoli florets.

Yield: 1 cup

1 cup cottage cheese
2 tablespoons milk
1 teaspoon dill weed
1 teaspoon dried chives
1 teaspoon celery seed

Combine all ingredients in a blender. Whirl until smooth. Refrigerate for several hours. Serve with raw vegetables.

• French Dressing •

This dressing is an excellent source of those critical omega-3 essential fatty acids.   *Yield: 3/4 cup*

1/2 teaspoon paprika
1/8 teaspoon dry mustard
1/2 cup pure canola, soy, or walnut oil
1/4 cup vinegar
1 tablespoon tomato paste
2 tablespoons concentrated frozen unsweetened apple or white grape juice,
    thawed; 3 packets Equal, Natra Taste, Sweet One, or Sweet'n Low;
    or a pinch of stevia
1 slice onion

Combine all ingredients except the onion in a covered container and shake well. Add onion and refrigerate. After 48 hours, remove the onion. Shake again before using. Use within one week.

• Italian Dressing •

This dressing is a great source of omega-3 essential fatty acids.
                                                              Yield: 1 1/3 cups

1 cup pure canola, soy, or walnut oil
1/3 cup vinegar
1/4 teaspoon dry mustard
1/4 teaspoon celery seed
1/8 teaspoon instant minced garlic
1/2 teaspoon salt
2 dashes pepper

Combine all ingredients in a covered jar and shake well. Refrigerate 24 hours before serving. Shake again before using. Use within one week.

• Barbecue Sauce •

Finding unsweetened barbecue sauces at grocery and health-food stores is nearly impossible. But don't give up on barbecue sauce yet! With this flavorful sauce, your kids will never even miss bottled barbecue sauces.

Yield: 2 cups

³/₄ cup chopped onion

¹/₂ cup pure canola, soy, or walnut oil

³/₄ cup sugar-free, honey-free tomato ketchup

³/₄ cup water

¹/₄ cup pure lemon juice

¹/₄ cup concentrated frozen unsweetened white grape or apple juice, thawed

2 tablespoons prepared mustard

2 teaspoons salt

¹/₂ teaspoon pepper

Cook onion in oil until soft. Add remaining ingredients. Simmer for 15 minutes. Refrigerate unused portion.

CAKES, PIES, COOKIES, AND BREADS

• Apple Cake •

Red or Golden Delicious apples, apple juice concentrate, and raisins provide all the sweetness you need in this cake.   *Yield: About 9 servings*

1¹/₂ cups unbleached flour; 1¹/₃ cups oat flour; or 1¹/₈ to 1¹/₄ cups rice flour

2 teaspoons baking soda

¹/₂ teaspoon salt

1 teaspoon cinnamon

1 teaspoon nutmeg

¹/₄ cup pure canola, soy, or walnut oil

¹/₄ cup butter or allowed margarine, softened

2 eggs (or equivalent in substitute)

¹/₄ cup water

¹/₄ cup frozen apple juice concentrate, thawed

1 teaspoon pure vanilla extract

4 cups peeled, cored, and chopped Delicious apples

1 cup Post Grape-Nuts

³/₄ cup raisins

Whipped Topping (see page 204)

In a large mixing bowl, combine flour, baking soda, salt, cinnamon, and nutmeg.

In another bowl, cream together oil, butter, and eggs. Beat in flour mixture. Stir in water, apple juice, and vanilla. Fold in apples, Grape-Nuts, and raisins. Pour into a greased and lightly floured 8-inch square pan. Bake at 350°F for 30 to 35 minutes, or until a toothpick inserted in the center comes out clean. Cool cake. Remove from pan. Top with Whipped Topping. Refrigerate leftovers.

• Apple or Pear Pie •

Use sweet apples such as Red Delicious or ripe sweet pears and you'll need no sugar or sweetener. This recipe is grand enough for guests.

Yield: 6 servings

2 pie crusts (see recipes on page 209)

6 cups peeled, cored, and sliced Delicious apples or pears

1 teaspoon cinnamon

¹/₈ teaspoon nutmeg

2 tablespoons cornstarch or flour or tapioca

2 tablespoons butter or allowed margarine

Arrange first pie crust in bottom of pie pan. Combine apples or pears with spices and cornstarch (or other allowed thickener) in bowl and toss lightly until thoroughly mixed. Place on the bottom crust. Dot with butter or margarine. Cover with second crust, seal, and cut slits to let steam escape. Bake for 35 to 40 minutes at 350°F until lightly browned with juices bubbly. Cool before serving.

• Pie Crusts •

Commercial pie crusts use lard, hydrogenated or partially hydrogenated oils, preservatives, and artificial color. You can easily make your own using "good" oils. There's even a wheat-free recipe for those sensitive to wheat.

• Basic Pie Crust •

Yield: 1 pie crust

1¹/₃ cup whole-wheat pastry flour
¹/₄ teaspoon salt
¹/₃ cup pure canola, soy, or walnut oil
2 tablespoons cold milk or ice cold water

Mix flour and salt together. Measure oil and liquid into a cup, mixing slightly. Add to the flour mixture. Stir until well mixed. Form the dough into a smooth ball. Place on a sheet of waxed paper and flatten a little. Cover with another sheet of waxed paper and roll out with a rolling pin to the desired size and thickness. Peel off top paper. Turn over into pie pan so remaining paper is on top. Carefully peel off paper. Fit into pan and press dough around the edges. If baking only the crust, prick in several spots with a fork. Bake for 10 to 12 minutes at 450°F, or until lightly browned.

• Nut Crust •

Yield: 1 pie crust

1 1/3 cups finely chopped walnuts
2 tablespoons butter, melted

Mix the nuts and butter together. Using the back of a spoon, press mixture against the sides and bottom of a pie pan. Bake at 350°F for 12 minutes. Cool before filling.

• Cinnamon Cookies •

These deliciously sweet cookies make a perfect holiday treat.

Yield: 24 2-inch cookies

1/2 cup regular butter
1/3 cup milk
1/2 teaspoon cinnamon
1 cup quick-cooking oats
1 cup Post Grape-Nuts
6 packets Equal, Natra Taste, Sweet One,
   or Sweet'n Low; or 1/16 teaspoon stevia
1 cup chopped dates

In a heavy saucepan, bring butter and milk to a boil. Remove from heat. Stir in remaining ingredients. Mix well. Form into 1-inch balls. Place on cookie sheet. Slightly flatten each. Chill. Keep refrigerated.

• Pumpkin Cookies •

These cookies are tasty, and nutritious too. You can feel good about offering a few of these a day to your child.   *Yield: 24 cookies*

¹/₂ cup butter, softened

¹/₂ cup pure canola, soy, or walnut oil

1 egg, beaten

¹/₂ cup frozen unsweetened concentrated orange juice, thawed

1 cup cooked pumpkin

1 teaspoon pure vanilla extract

1¹/₂ cups whole-wheat pastry flour

¹/₂ teaspoon baking soda

¹/₂ teaspoon baking powder

1 teaspoon cinnamon

¹/₄ teaspoon nutmeg

1 teaspoon ginger

¹/₂ cup chopped dates

¹/₂ cup walnuts

¹/₄ cup ground flaxseed

In a large bowl, mix together butter, oil, egg, orange juice, pumpkin, and vanilla. In a separate large bowl, combine remaining ingredients. Add wet ingredients to dry ingredients. Mix well. Drop tablespoonsful of batter onto an ungreased cookie sheet. Bake at 350°F for 15 minutes. Remove from cookie sheet and let cool on a wire rack.

• Vanilla Cookies •

These cookies are always a crowd favorite. No one will even notice that there's no sugar. *Yield: 24 cookies*

1³/₄ cups whole-wheat pastry flour

1¹/₂ teaspoons baking powder

¹/₄ teaspoon salt

¹/₂ cup chopped dates

¹/₂ cup chopped walnuts

*¹/₂ cup unsweetened concentrated white grape juice or
   concentrated apple juice*
¹/₄ cup butter, softened
¹/₄ cup pure canola, soy, or walnut oil
1 egg, beaten
1 teaspoon pure vanilla extract

In a large bowl, mix together flour, baking powder, salt, dates, and walnuts. In a medium bowl, mix together remaining ingredients. Add wet ingredients to dry and mix well. Drop teaspoonfuls of batter onto an ungreased baking sheet. Bake at 350°F for 10 to 12 minutes. Cool on wire rack.

• Oatmeal Cookies •

Raisins and concentrated apple juice provide all the sweetness these cookies need. The oatmeal and whole-wheat pastry flour are both nutritious.   *Yield: 24 cookies*

³/₄ cup whole-wheat pastry flour
1 teaspoon cinnamon
¹/₂ teaspoon baking soda
¹/₂ teaspoon salt
1¹/₂ cups rolled oats
¹/₂ cup raisins
¹/₂ cup butter, softened
¹/₂ cup concentrated frozen apple juice, thawed
1 egg, beaten
1 teaspoon pure vanilla extract

In a large bowl, mix together flour, cinnamon, baking soda, salt, oats, and raisins. In another bowl, beat together butter, apple juice, egg, and vanilla. Add wet ingredients to dry and mix well. Drop teaspoonfuls of batter onto an ungreased baking sheet and bake at 350°F for about 10 minutes. Remove from sheet and cool on wire rack.

• Thumbprint Cookies •

Your children will enjoy helping you make these fun-to-make cookies.

Yield: 15 cookies

1/2 cup butter, softened
1 egg
1/2 teaspoon pure vanilla extract
1 1/4 to 1 3/8 cups unbleached flour or whole-wheat pastry flour
1/2 cup finely chopped walnuts
All-fruit jam or jelly

Beat together butter, egg, vanilla, and enough flour so dough is no longer sticky. Work in nuts. Chill until firm enough to shape. Roll into balls. Place on ungreased cookie sheet. Dip your thumb in flour and press down firmly in the middle of each cookie. Bake at 350°F for about 15 minutes or until golden brown on the bottoms. Remove from oven. Cool. Fill hollows with jam or jelly. Keep refrigerated.

• Apricot Egg Replacer •

If your child is sensitive to eggs, you can use this substitute in cookies, muffins, meat loaf, cakes, and quick breads to help bind the ingredients together while adding some sweetness.

Yield: 1 1/4 cups

6 ounces sun-dried apricots
1 1/2 cups water

Boil apricots in water until soft. Cool. Puree in blender. Keep refrigerated in a covered container. Use 2 tablespoons apricot egg replacer for each egg called for in a recipe. Add an extra ½ teaspoon baking powder per egg to make batter rise in appropriate recipes.

• Pumpkin Pie •

Your family will enjoy this holiday favorite any time of the year. The pumpkin is an excellent source of vitamin A (as beta-carotene). Rice milk can be used instead of cow's milk if your child is milk-sensitive.

Yield: 1 8- or 9-inch pie (6 servings)

1³/4 cups (1 15-ounce can) cooked pumpkin

¼ cup concentrated frozen unsweetened white grape juice, thawed

2 eggs, beaten

½ teaspoon salt

¼ teaspoon nutmeg

1 teaspoon cinnamon

½ teaspoon ginger

1¼ cups milk or Enriched Rice Dream Milk

1 unbaked pie crust (see recipe on page 209)

In a large bowl, beat together all ingredients and pour into the pie crust. Bake at 425°F for 15 minutes. Reduce heat to 350°F. Bake for 40 to 50 minutes. Pie is done when knife inserted in center comes out clean. Serve immediately or chill. Refrigerate leftovers.

• Wheat Bread •

Most commercial bread contains corn sweeteners or sugar, partially hydrogenated vegetable oil, and preservatives. If you're fortunate enough to have a bread maker, making your own bread will be a snap. If you don't own a bread maker, the following recipe is quick and easy and doesn't require kneading.

Yield: 2 loaves

¼ cup butter or allowed margarine

3 cups warm water

1 tablespoon salt

3 packages dry yeast

3 cups whole-wheat flour

2½ to 2¾ cups unbleached flour

Combine butter, 2 cups water, and salt. Dissolve yeast in 1 cup warm water. Combine with butter mixture. Stir in whole-wheat flour and half the white flour. Beat with an electric mixer for 2 minutes. Add remaining white flour and stir well, using a heavy spoon. Pour into two well-greased 9×5-inch loaf pans. Cover and let rise in a warm place for about 45 minutes or until doubled in bulk. Bake for 1 hour at 400°F. If bottom of loaf pan sounds hollow when tapped, bread is done. Remove from pans. Let loaves cool thoroughly on a wire rack.

FRUIT SNACKS, GELATINS, AND FROZEN TREATS

• Banana Salad •

Not only is this treat delicious, it's nutritious. It could almost serve as a meal—the banana is a serving of fruit, and the nut butter and walnuts are a serving of protein.   *Yield: 1 serving*

1 banana

1 tablespoon natural peanut butter or almond butter

1 tablespoon chopped walnuts

1 lettuce leaf

Slice banana into fourths and put in a bowl. Coat banana with a layer of nut butter. Sprinkle with chopped walnuts. Serve on a lettuce leaf.

• Fruit Leather •

Commercial fruit roll-ups snacks are loaded with sugar, corn syrup, and artificial colors, but no fruit! These are healthy—and tasty—alternatives. Do remember, though, that these treats are high in natural sweeteners, so use them sparingly.   *Yield: 12 pieces*

5 or 6 large pieces ripe, sweet-tasting fruit (apples, peaches, pears, plums, bananas, apricots, or nectarines)

Wash fruit thoroughly. Remove skin. Cut into chunks and blend on high speed until smooth. Lightly oil an 11×17-inch shallow baking pan. Pour fruit onto the pan and spread evenly. Put into the oven at 170°F, and leave the door ajar to let moisture escape. Leave in the oven until the fruit has dried evenly all over and can be lifted from the pan—about 1 to 2 hours. Cut into pieces and wrap in waxed paper.

• Fruit Juice Gelatin •

This dessert makes an easy, delicious, colorful, and nutritious substitute for flavored gelatins such as Jell-O—and it contains no artificial colors or flavors.   *Yield: 4 servings*

1 envelope unflavored gelatin
2 cups unsweetened grape, orange, pineapple, or cherry-cranberry juice
2 packets Equal, Natra Taste, Sweet One, or Sweet'n Low (optional)
1½ cups crushed unsweetened pineapple (canned), pears, orange sections, grapefruit sections, grapes, etc.

In a small saucepan soften gelatin in ¼ cup fruit juice. Stir over low heat until gelatin dissolves completely. Add gelatin to remaining juice. Stir in sweetener. Chill until partially set. Fold in unsweetened fruits. Chill until firm.

• Fruit Juice Ice Pops •

Easy and nutritious—and no added sugar and artificial colors or flavors.

Yield: 8 ice pops

2 cups unsweetened grape, orange, or apple juice
1 or 2 packets Equal, Natra Taste, Sweet One, or Sweet'n Low (optional)

Mix the juice and sweetener together. Pour into eight 3-ounce paper cups (or ice-pop molds). Insert a plastic spoon in the middle of each. Freeze until firm. Unmold by briefly dipping each cup in hot water.

• Melon Icc Pops •

These healthy, naturally sweet ice pops are also free of artificial colors and flavors that are found in most commercial ice pops.   *Yield: 4 servings*

2 cups small watermelon, cantaloupe, or honeydew melon cubes
   (seeds discarded)

In a blender, process melon cubes until smooth. Pour into ice pop molds or small Dixie cups. Insert a spoon to serve as a handle. Freeze until firm.

• Orange or Pineapple Ice Cream •

If your child can tolerate milk and oranges or pineapples but not artificial sweeteners, he'll love this ice cream.   *Yield: 1 pint*

1 pint half-and-half
3/4 cup unsweetened frozen orange juice or pineapple concentrate, thawed
2 tablespoons grated orange rind

Combine all ingredients. Process according to manufacturer's directions in an ice cream maker, or pour into a shallow pan, cover, and freeze until almost firm. Place in a large, chilled mixing bowl and beat with an electric mixer until smooth. Return to pan. Cover tightly and freeze until firm.

• Orange or Grape Snow •

This treat makes a nutritious milk-free frozen dessert or snack.

Yield: 4 servings

¾ cup frozen orange or grape juice concentrate, thawed
1 cup water

Combine ingredients. Pour into an ice cube tray with separator. Freeze until firm. Remove cubes from tray. Grind in food processor until finely grated. Put snow into four bowls and serve immediately.

• Strawberry Soft Serve •

My children always enjoyed this frozen dessert. If you like, you can substitute frozen peaches or blueberries for the strawberries.

Yield: 4 servings

1 20-ounce package frozen unsweetened strawberries
1 cup half-and-half, 2-percent milk, Enriched Rice Dream Milk, or soymilk
¼ cup frozen concentrated unsweetened orange or white grape juice, thawed;
* or 4 packets Equal, Natra Taste, Sweet One, or Sweet'n Low*

Place all ingredients in blender. Blend until smooth. Serve immediately.

BEVERAGES

• Carob Milk •

Commercial chocolate milk is full of sugar and sometimes artificial colors and flavors. In addition, many children with ADHD are sensitive to chocolate. Carob powder makes a great chocolate substitute.

Yield: 1 8-ounce serving

8 ounces cold skim or 2-percent milk
1 tablespoon carob powder
1 packet Equal, Natra Taste, Sweet One, or Sweet'n Low;
*   or a pinch of stevia*
⅛ teaspoon pure vanilla extract

Mix together all ingredients.

• Fruit Juice Pop •

Soda pop that's nutritious? Try this one.   *Yield: 1 serving*

4 ounces pure unsweetened grape, orange, or pineapple juice
4 ounces soda water or Perrier water

Combine juice and soda water. Serve over ice cubes.

• Fruit Smoothies •

If you have trouble getting your child to eat breakfast, you can try this fruit drink. It is easy and nutritious. If your child is sensitive to milk, you can use rice or soymilk. Choose brands that are enriched with calcium and vitamin D. The flaxseed adds omega-3 fatty acids. If you choose rice milk for this recipe, serve it with a food source of protein, as rice milk contains little protein.   *Yield: 1 serving*

6 ounces low-fat milk, Enriched Rice Dream Milk, or soymilk
1 tablespoon frozen unsweetened white grape juice concentrate, thawed
1 cup frozen strawberries
1 tablespoon ground flaxseed
1 teaspoon pure vanilla extract (optional)

Combine all ingredients in a blender. Whirl until smooth. Serve immediately.

• Apple Lemonade •

This is a delicious, nutritious version of the old-time favorite drink without sugar or artificial sweeteners.   *Yield: 2 servings*

2 cups pure, unsweetened apple juice
4 tablespoons pure lemon juice

Combine juices. Chill. Serve over ice.

• Strawberry Slush •

Your child should enjoy this cool beverage on a hot summer day.

Yield: 4 servings

1 20-ounce package frozen unsweetened strawberries
¼ cup frozen unsweetened white grape juice concentrate, thawed;

or 4 packets Equal, Natra Taste, Sweet One, or Sweet'n Low;
or a pinch of stevia
3 cups (24 ounces) chilled club soda

In a blender, whirl frozen strawberries, sweetener, and half the club soda until smooth. Divide slush among four large glasses. Add remaining soda and stir well. Serve immediately.

CONCLUSION

By now you've identified potential pieces to your child's hyperactivity jigsaw puzzle. For one child, the pieces might be food sensitivities (milk, chocolate, artificial colors) and essential fatty acid deficiencies. For another child, identifying food sensitivities (milk and wheat), treating yeast sensitivities, and avoiding sugar may change the child's life. For another child, identifying and treating a thyroid hormone deficiency may produce amazing results. And for every child, eating a nutritious diet is a major piece in his puzzle.

Helping a child with ADD/ADHD should be a team effort. If your child is taking medication, he should be supervised closely by his pediatrician or psychiatrist. If he improves using the methods in this book, then share the information with your doctor and ask for her help in adjusting or stopping medication. Don't try to do this on your own.

A child psychologist skilled in helping children with ADHD may be another member of the team. If you're spending all your time yelling at your child, then a counselor can help you choose effective ways to manage your child. Parenting classes may give you new approaches to child rearing that will really work. It's not that you're a "bad" parent, it's just that parenting a child with ADHD requires the patience of a saint! You may also find parent support classes helpful. Children and Adults with Attention Deficit Disorder (CHADD) is a national support group with chapters all over the country. However, the main approach to treating ADD that it supports is medication. The Feingold Association is a support group for parents of children with ADD. It, too, is a national group with chapters in many cities. It supports the use of diet as a primary way to help children with ADHD. (See Appendix C for the Internet sites for CHADD and the Feingold Association.) A support group for your child, such as CHADD, might help him gain social skills, exercise self-control, and raise self-esteem.

Another source of help can be your child's school. Ask his teacher to assist your child in watching his diet. She can tell you ahead of time if there are parties or celebrations coming up so you can send appropriate foods for your child, or perhaps you could keep cookies appropriate for your child in the nurse's freezer for special occasions. Other members of the team at school include the principal, speech therapists, occupational therapists, special-education teachers, and school psychologists. They will help your child's teacher adopt the best educational strategies and provide special services.

Perhaps someday a new member of the team will routinely include a nutritionist who is knowledgeable about biological factors in ADHD. I recently attended school conferences for two children in an attempt to set up individual education plans tailored toward these children. Everyone was very interested in the biological factors important for these children.

Of course, in dire situations—if your child's school is ready to expel him, if your spouse is threatening to leave home, or if your child is irritable, angry, depressed, and frustrated—then a trial of stimulant medication might be the answer, at least for now. In such cases, medication may provide short-term improvement. In the long run, however, doesn't it make more sense to at least look for pieces of his hyperactivity puzzle?

If your child is already on medication and it has helped his inattention and hyperactivity, you can continue the medicine while you look for better answers. If your child has never tried medication and his problems are manageable, then you can now look for pieces of his hyperactivity puzzle. For the child who's tried various medications that didn't help or caused side effects, you'll want to try the approaches discussed in this book.

You may have been told by your doctor, "There is no cure for ADHD. Stimulant medication is the only solution." In a letter to the editor in *U.S. News & World Report*, Leo Galland, M.D., pointed out that in a study of food sensitivities in children with severe ADHD, one-half of the children studied improved substantially on the few-foods diet and symptoms disappeared in a third of the children.[1] Dr. Galland commented, "If that isn't a 'cure,' then what is?"

The study of the relationship of nutritional factors to behavior and learning is in its infancy. There is a great need for more well-designed studies on treatment alternatives for ADHD. Eugene Arnold, M.D., professor emeritus of psychiatry at Ohio State University, has studied the medical literature to look for such alternatives. He concluded, "Most of the alternatives have been relatively neglected by most mainstream investigators and by peer-reviewed funding, despite the fact that some of them could be relatively cheaply tested."[2]

C. K. Conners, a prominent researcher in the ADD/ADHD community, has written:

> *Even if a child is eating a reasonably well-balanced diet, there are still many questions needing answers for any specific child: Which specific foods aggravate symptoms and should be removed? Does adding vitamin and mineral supplements improve my child's brain function? Which carbohydrates does my child react to most strongly? If I remove artificial flavors and colors, will it help my child's irritability and sleep problems? And so on. For these questions, parents cannot wait while the government funds more studies and scientists continue to wrangle. Each parent must become a scientific observer—objective, systematic, and curious about their own infants and school children.*[3]

So there you have it. Twelve ways to play detective and help your hyperactive child without drugs. Good luck and best wishes.

APPENDIX A.
SCIENTIFIC STUDIES FOR
YOU AND YOUR DOCTOR

I recently received an e-mail from a Canadian psychiatrist who concluded, "I am sorry to disappoint you. There is no other alternative that showed proof of its efficacy in ADHD but the stimulants." Evidently, he hasn't had time to read the latest research. He might be surprised that well-controlled studies have been reported in such prestigious medical journals as *The Lancet, Annals of Allergy, Pediatrics, Journal of Pediatrics*, and others. There have been a number of studies since the mid-1980s that clearly demonstrate that there are alternatives to stimulant drugs for many children with ADHD. Ask your librarian to order these scientific articles for you on Interlibrary Loan. Then share copies with your doctor. Perhaps that will encourage her to become interested in helping your child and other children in her practice using this latest research.

ADHD and Sensitivies to Foods and Food Additives

Egger, J. "Controlled Trial of Oligoantigenic Treatment in the Hyper-kinetic Syndrome." *Lancet* 1 (March 9, 1985): 540–45.

Summary: Seventy-six children were treated with a diet of only a few foods—those researchers thought were least likely to cause reactions. Sixty-two children improved on this diet. Artificial colors and preservatives were the most common culprits (79 percent), but no child was sensitive to these alone. Other common foods that caused reactions were soy (72 percent), milk (64 percent), chocolate (58 percent), wheat (49 percent), and sugar (16 percent). (Not every child was challenged with every food.) Twenty-eight of these children took part in a double-blind, crossover, placebo-controlled trial in which suspected foods were returned to the diet one at a time. Suspected food caused significantly more behavioral problems and physical complaints than the control foods.

Conclusion: "Further work along these lines is clearly necessary."

Kaplan, B. "Dietary Replacement in Preschool-Aged Hyperactive Boys." *Pediatrics* 83 (1989): 7–17.

Summary: Twenty-four hyperactive boys were studied while eating foods that were provided by the researchers. The experimental diet eliminated artificial colors and flavors, chocolate, monosodium glutamate, preservatives, caffeine, and any food a family suspected. The diet was low in sugar and was dairy-free if the family suspected cow's milk. More than half the subjects improved on this diet with negligible improvement while eating a placebo diet.

Conclusion: "These results suggest that pediatricians and other practitioners might consider dietary modifications worth trying, particularly in younger children."

Carter, C. M. "Effects of a Few Foods Diet in Attention-Deficit Disorder." *Archives of Diseases of Childhood* 69 (1993): 564–68.

Summary: Seventy-eight hyperactive children were placed on a few-foods elimination diet. Fifty-nine (76 percent) improved. In an open trial, the most common culprits included additive-containing foods (70 percent), chocolate (64 percent), cow's milk (64 percent), oranges (57 percent), and cheese (45 percent). Nineteen of these children took part in placebo-controlled, double-blind challenges of suspected foods. The suspected foods caused significantly more changes in behavior than foods that acted as placebos.

Conclusion: "Clinicians should give weight to the accounts of parents and consider this treatment in selected children with a suggestive medical history."

Boris, M. "Foods and Additives Are Common Causes of the Attention Deficit Hyperactive Disorder in Children." *Annals of Allergy* 72 (1994): 462–68.

Summary: Twenty-six children with ADHD completed a two-week open elimination diet that avoided dairy products, wheat, corn, yeast, soy, citrus, egg, chocolate, peanuts, artificial colors, and preservatives. Nineteen of the twenty-six children (73 percent) improved on this diet. Seventy-nine percent of these children had a history of allergy. In a double-blind, controlled study, suspected foods were disguised in other foods and behaviors noted. Suspected foods caused significantly more behavioral changes than placebo.

Conclusion: "Dietary factors may play a significant role in the etiology of the majority of children with ADHD."

Rowe, K., and K. Rowe. "Synthetic Food Coloring and Behavior: A Dose Response Effect in a Double-Blind, Placebo-Controlled, Repeated-Measures Study." *Journal of Pediatrics* 125 (1994): 691–98.

Summary: Two hundred children whose parents suspected that they reacted to various foods were enrolled in a six-week open trial of a diet free of artificial food colors. One hundred and fifty children showed improved behavior on the diet and were worse when the colorings were added back to their diets. Parents noted that when their children ate foods with food dyes they exhibited more irritability, restlessness, and sleep problems. Next, thirty-four children completed a double-blind, placebo-controlled trial. For twenty-one days, the children took either a placebo (lactose) or tartrazine (FD&C yellow No. 5) buried in an inner capsule placed in a capsule with lactose. Both supplements looked identical. Six different doses of the yellow dye were chosen. Twenty-four children were clear reactors. Significant reactions were noted with every dose of the yellow coloring, and the larger the dose, the more prolonged the reaction.

Conclusion: "Behavioral changes in irritability, restlessness, and sleep disturbances are associated with the ingestion of tartrazine in some children. A dose response effect was observed."

Food Sensitivities and Ear Infections

Hagerman, R. J., and A. R. Falkenstein. "An Association Between Recurrent Otitis Media in Infancy and Later Hyperactivity." *Clinical Pediatrics* (May 1987): 253–57.

Summary: Sixty-seven children were referred for evaluation because of failure in school. Every child had specific learning problems, and twenty-seven were hyperactive. More than 69 percent had had more than ten ear infections, while 94 percent had had three or more.

Conclusion: "The authors have found a correlation between an increasing number of otitis infections and the severity of hyperactivity when investigating a population of hyperactive and non-hyperactive children who exhibited failure in school. Further investigation is necessary to evaluate etiologic aspects of this association."

Nsouli, T. M., et al. "Role of Food Allergy in Serous Otitis Media." *Annals of Allergy* 73 (1994): 215–19.

Summary: One hundred four children with recurrent ear infections were evaluated for food allergy. Patients who were allergic to specific foods followed a diet free of these foods for sixteen weeks. An open food challenge was given for each suspected food. Seventy-eight percent of the children developed symptoms of ear infections again. The most common offending foods were cow's milk, wheat, egg, peanut, soy, corn, and orange. Most children were sensitive to two to four foods.

Conclusion: "The possibility of food allergy should be considered in all pediatric patients with recurrent serous otitis media and a diligent search for the putative food allergens made for proper diagnosis and therapeutic intervention."

Food Sensitivities and Bed Wetting and Migraine Headaches

Robson, W. L., et al. "Enuresis in Children with Attention-Deficit Hyperactivity Disorder." *Southern Medical Journal* 90 (1997): 503–5.

Summary: Enuresis (involuntary urination) affects 10 percent of five-year-old children and 5 percent of ten-year-olds. Two hundred patients with ADHD ages six to fourteen were identified by researchers from records at a developmental pediatric clinic. Parents were asked to complete questionnaires about night and day enuresis in their children. Parents of children with normal behavior completed the same questionnaires.

Conclusion: "In our case-control study, a significant association was found between ADHD and nocturnal and diurnal enuresis in children at the age of six years. Physicians who treat patients with ADHD should be aware of this finding and should routinely inquire about the presence of enuresis."

Egger, J., et al. "Effect of Diet Treatment on Enuresis in Children with Migraine or Hyperkinetic Behavior." *Clinical Pediatrics* (1992): 302–7.

Summary: Twenty-one children who had migraine headaches and/or ADHD also suffered from nightly and/or daily wetting. These children were treated with a few-foods diet of hypoallergenic foods. On the diet, twelve children stopped wetting and four others improved. When various foods were returned to the diet, the children had wetting problems again. Nine children were selected to participate in a double-blind study. Six children had wetting with incriminated foods and none reacted to the placebo. The most common foods provoking wetting were chocolate, oranges, yellow dye, and milk.

Conclusion: "Enuresis in food-induced migraine and/or behavior disorder seems to respond, in some patients, to avoidance of provoking foods."

Egger, J. "Oligoantigenic Diet Treatment of Children with Epilepsy and Migraine," *Journal of Pediatrics* 114 (1989): 51–58.

Summary: Doctors studied forty-five children who had epilepsy and also had headaches and abdominal pains or ADHD. On a few-foods diet of hypoallergenic foods twenty-five of the children no longer had seizures while eleven showed fewer seizures. When various foods were added back to the diet, seizures recurred. In double-blind studies, symptoms recurred in fifteen of sixteen children. The most common symptom-provoking foods were milk, citrus foods, wheat, yellow dye, and eggs. Interestingly, when eighteen different children with seizures but without the other symptoms were given the few-foods diet, none improved.

Conclusion: "We have seen response to diet in children who have both epilepsy and migraine, so this treatment might apply only to a minority of epileptic children. However, we believe that it deserves a trial in some patients with drug-resistant epilepsy and migraine."

Egger, J. "Is Migraine Food Allergy?" *Lancet* 8355 (1983): 865–68.

Summary: Ninety-three percent of eighty-eight children who suffered from severe and frequent migraine headaches improved on a few-foods diet of hypoallergenic foods. Seventy-eight children recovered completely, four improved greatly, and six did not improve. Foods were returned to the diet one per week and reactions noted. Next, a double-blind, placebo-controlled study was conducted with forty of the children. All but eight relapsed when offending foods were added back to the diet disguised in other foods. The most common headache-provoking foods included milk, chocolate, oranges, wheat, benzoic acid, tomato, and yellow dye (tartrazine).

Conclusion: "This trial showed that most children with severe frequent migraine recover on an appropriate diet, and that so many foods can provoke attacks that any food or combination of foods may be the cause."

APPENDIX B.

JIMMY'S COMMON FOODS
ELIMINATION DIET
AND DIARY

Jimmy suffered from ADHD, and his doctor recommended Ritalin. Jimmy's mother did not like the idea of his taking medication for the rest of his life, so she looked into nutritional therapy options. She learned about the Common Foods Elimination Diet and decided to give it a try. Jimmy's elimination diet avoided sugar, chocolate, milk, eggs, corn, wheat, rye, citrus fruits (oranges, grapefruits, lemons, tangerines, limes), sugar, and legumes (soy, peas, beans, peanuts), as well as artificial colors and flavors and preservatives—those foods he ate most often. He avoided all these foods and food additives for a week, until he felt and acted better for a few days. Then, one day at a time, his mother reintroduced each food and noted Jimmy's behavioral and physical symptoms. She kept a diary of Jimmy's daily menus and his general behavior. Jimmy felt worse the first few days, as often happens, so don't be surprised if that happens to your child. Hang in there, persevere!

Following is a copy of the diary Jimmy's mom kept of Jimmy's daily menus and behavior throughout the diet to serve as a model for you to follow.

Day 1

MEAL	FOODS	DIARY OF REACTIONS
Breakfast	Broiled hamburger, fried potatoes in pure safflower oil, unsweetened applesauce, unsweetened pineapple juice	Really hyper. Uncooperative. Won't get dressed. Won't sit down to eat.
Snack	Banana, unprocessed almonds	
Lunch	Plain hamburger with mustard, allowed potato chips (no preservatives, fried in pure safflower oil), fresh sliced pear, carrot sticks, unsweetened grape juice	Hyper. Irritable. Complains that he misses all his favorite foods.
Snack	Walnuts, carrots, and celery sticks	
Dinner	Baked chicken, rice, cooked carrots, tossed salad with allowed dressing, fresh sliced peach	Hyper. Can't sit down to eat. Crying. Depressed. Says he hates this diet.
Snack	Rice cakes with almond butter	Won't settle down to go to bed. Hyper. Won't brush teeth. Uncooperative.

Day 2

Breakfast	Oatmeal with Rice Dream Milk, broiled pork chop, fresh sliced peach, unsweetened grape juice	Won't sit down to eat. All over the place. Crying over everything.
Snack	Unprocessed almonds, grapes	
Lunch	Leftover cold baked chicken, allowed potato chips, carrot sticks, tomato juice	Hyper. Irritable. Whines constantly.
Snack	Almond butter on celery	

| Dinner | Allowed spaghetti sauce on rice, tossed salad with allowed dressing, steamed broccoli, watermelon, ice water | Extremely hyper. He hates this diet, and so do I!!! |
| Snack | Walnuts, fresh sliced pear | Went to bed rather easily. |

Day 3

Breakfast	Broiled homemade sausage patty, oatmeal with Enriched Rice Dream Milk, cantaloupe, pineapple juice	Seems a little better. Is there really hope?
Snack	Celery with cashew butter	
Lunch	Tuna salad with allowed mayonnaise, rice cake, carrot sticks, fresh sliced pear, ice water	Better morning. Not so hyper.
Snack	Cold leftover baked chicken, peeled apple	
Dinner	Broiled fish, baked sweet potato, rice, fruit cup of allowed fruits, unsweetened pineapple juice	Sat down to eat dinner— a first! Calmer.
Snack	Kiwi slices, raw cashews	Went to bed well. Good day!!

Day 4

Breakfast	Broiled lamb chop, rice cake with clarified butter, banana, ice water	Slept well. Calmer. Cooperative. Like a different child.
Snack	Sunflower seeds, unsweetened pineapple juice	
Lunch	Tuna salad on rice cake, carrots, celery sticks, sliced fresh peach, unsweetened grape juice	Excellent morning.
Snack	Cashew butter on rice cake with allowed all-fruit preserves	

| Dinner | Beef stew thickened with allowed starch, rice, cooked carrots, watermelon | Doing great. Looks and acts like he feels better. |
| Snack | Almond butter on rice cake, grapes | Went to bed so easily. |

Day 5

| Repeated menus for Day 1. | | Did well all day. Happy. Calm. Cooperative. Full of hugs and kisses. |

Day 6

| Repeated menus for Day 2. | | Good day. |

Day 7

| Repeated menus for Day 3. | | Good day. |

Day 8—Reintroduce *Eggs*

Breakfast	*Boiled egg*, fried potatoes, unsweetened applesauce, unsweetened pineapple juice	Doing well.
Snack	Apple, *hard-boiled egg*	
Lunch	Egg salad on rice cake, allowed potato chips, carrot sticks, unsweetened pineapple chunks	Doing well.

Snack	Cashew butter on celery, carrot sticks, *hard-boiled egg*	
Dinner	Baked chicken, *hard-boiled egg*, rice, steamed broccoli, banana	Continues to do well.
Snack	Rice cakes with almond butter	Not sensitive to eggs!

Day 9—Reintroduce *Sugar*

Breakfast	Oatmeal with *sugar*, Enriched Rice Dream Milk, broiled pork chop, banana, grape juice with *sugar* added	Okay. Calm.
Snack	Raw almonds, grape juice with sugar added	Crying. Whining. More hyper.
Lunch	Cold leftover baked chicken, fresh grapes, allowed potato chips, ice water	Definitely more emotional and hyper. *Stop sugar!*
Snack	Almond butter on celery.	Still all wound up. Can't sit still.
Dinner	Allowed spaghetti sauce on rice, tossed salad with allowed dressing, cooked carrots, watermelon, ice water	Crying, irritable.
Snack	Walnuts, unsweetened grape juice	Awful all day. Glad day is over.

Day 10—Reintroduce *Corn*

Breakfast	*Corn on the cob*, homemade sausage patty, banana, unsweetened pineapple juice	Seems good this morning.
Snack	*Air popped popcorn*, sliced kiwi	Okay.
Lunch	Corn on the cob, leftover baked chicken, carrot sticks, apple, tomato juice	Continues to do well.
Snack	*Popcorn*, celery with almond butter	

Dinner	*Corn on the cob*, baked fish, steamed asparagus, fruit cup of allowed fruits, tomato juice	Okay.
Snack	*Popcorn*, apple juice	Excellent day. Not sensitive to corn!

Day 11—Reintroduce *Wheat*

Breakfast	*Whole-wheat* pancakes (no milk, sugar, or eggs) with allowed all-fruit preserves, broiled lamb chop, apple, grapes	Doing well.
Snack	Leftover pancake with almond butter, apple juice	
Lunch	*Cream of Wheat* with Rice Dream Milk, fresh sliced peach, cold broiled lamb chop, unsweetened grape juice	Seems fine.
Snack	*Leftover pancake* with almond butter, banana	
Dinner	Allowed spaghetti sauce on cooked *spaghetti*, fruit cup of allowed fruits	Doing well.
Snack	Almond butter on celery	Good day. Wheat seems okay.

Day 12—Reintroduce *Peanuts*

Breakfast	Rice cake with *natural peanut butter*, homemade sausage patty, fried potatoes in pure safflower oil, unsweetened applesauce, ice water	Okay. Good night.
Snack	*Unprocessed peanuts*, apple	
Lunch	*Natural peanut butter* on rice cake with all-fruit preserves, allowed potato chips, carrot sticks, tomato juice	Fine.
Snack	Natural peanut butter on carrots and celery sticks	

Dinner	Baked chicken, steamed broccoli, tossed salad with allowed dressing, watermelon and cantaloupe balls, ice water	Doing well.
Snack	*Unprocessed peanuts*, apple juice	Good day. Not sensitive to peanuts. Hooray!

Day 13—Reintroduce *Oranges*

Breakfast	Oatmeal with Rice Dream Milk, broiled pork chop, *fresh orange sections, fresh-squeezed orange juice*	Calm, happy. Had a good night.
Snack	*Fresh-squeezed orange juice,* unprocessed almonds	
Lunch	Cold leftover chicken, baked potato with allowed margarine, cooked carrots, fresh-squeezed orange juice	No changes.
Snack	*Fresh-squeezed orange juice*, almond butter on celery	
Dinner	Allowed spaghetti sauce on rice, tossed salad with allowed dressing, sliced kiwi	Doing well.
Snack	*Fresh orange sections*, unprocessed almonds	Good day. Oranges are not a problem.

Day 14—Reintroduce *Chocolate*

Breakfast	Sausage patty, rice cake with allowed margarine, fresh sliced peach, unsweetened pineapple juice, piece of unsweetened *chocolate*	Okay this morning.
Snack	Rice cake with almond butter, piece of unsweetened *chocolate*	Irritable, crying.
Lunch	Leftover cold chicken, allowed potato chips, carrot sticks, apple, unsweetened grape juice	Runny nose. Dark circles under eyes. Depressed. Crying. *Stop chocolate!*
Snack	Unsweetened pineapple chunks, unprocessed almonds	

| Dinner | Baked fish, baked sweet potato, steamed asparagus, watermelon cubes, ice water | Still depressed. Very irritable. |
| Snack | Unprocessed cashews, grapes | Still grumpy. Glad day is over. |

Day 15—Reintroduce *Food Colorings*

Breakfast	Broiled hamburger, fried potatoes, unsweetened applesauce, mixed all McCormick's (or French's) *food colorings* together and added ½ teaspoon of mixture to unsweetened grape juice.	Seems better. Had a good night.
Snack	Rice cake with almond butter, grapes	Extremely hyper. Headache. Legs ache. *Stop colorings!*
Lunch	Tuna salad on rice cake, carrot and celery sticks, allowed potato chips, grapes, ice water	Still awful. Can't believe reaction to colorings.
Snack	Leftover cold chicken, unsweetened grape juice	
Dinner	Beef stew, rice, fruit cup of allowed fruits	Legs and head still ache. Irritable.
Snack	Almond butter on rice cake, grapes	Wet bed.

Day 16—Reintroduce *Milk*

Breakfast	Broiled sausage patty, fried potatoes, unsweetened applesauce, *milk*	Hurrah! Last day. Jimmy seems better today.
Snack	Unprocessed cashews, *milk*	More hyper? Irritable?
Lunch	Broiled hamburger with allowed ketchup, allowed potato chips, carrot sticks, unsweetened grape juice	Dark circles under eyes. Nose running. Legs ache. *Stop milk!*
Snack	Cashew butter on celery, grapes	

Dinner	Baked chicken, baked potato with allowed margarine, cooked carrots, cantaloupe and watermelon cubes, ice water	
Snack	Unprocessed almonds, sliced kiwi	Nose is still running. Looks pale and washed out.

Conclusions: Jimmy is sensitive to sugar, chocolate, artificial colors, and milk. He will need to take a calcium supplement as long as he is avoiding dairy products.

Plan: Add safe foods (eggs, corn, wheat, oranges, and peanuts) back to diet. Avoid the foods and colorings Jimmy reacted to for several months. Then reintroduce each in a small amount once or twice a week if tolerated. Still to be reintroduced and tested (one per day) are rye, other citrus fruits, and other legumes (soy, beans, peas).

•

Keep track of the foods your child eats at each meal. You might want to reward him in this way: Every time he eats the allowed foods, he earns a star. At the end of each day, if he has earned at least six stars, he earns a small prize. At the end of two weeks, if he hasn't cheated on his diet, he earns a big prize. You will deserve one too. After the diet is completed, treat yourself to new clothes, a movie, lunch with friends—something you'll look forward to. Of course, the biggest reward of all would be a marked improvement in your child's behavior.

APPENDIX C.

Books

Amen, A. J., S. Johnson, D. G. Amen. *A Teenager's Guide to A.D.D.* Fairfield, CA: MindWorks Press, 1996. This book is written for teenagers who have ADD. This book will help the teenager understand ADD and how to get help at home, at school, and with peers. School survival skills will be especially helpful.

Baker, S. M. *Detoxification and Healing.* New Canaan, CT: Keats, 1997. Although this book doesn't address the specific problems of children with ADHD, its approaches to optimal health apply to everyone. You'll find it fascinating and informative.

Barkley, R. A. *Attention-Deficit Hyperactivity Disorder: A Handbook for Diagnosis and Treatment.* New York: Guilford Press, 1998. This is an interesting book for professionals and parents by a nationally renowned researcher. It explores in depth the etiologies of ADHD, diagnosis, and treatment.

Block, M. A. *No More Ritalin*. New York: Kensington Press, 1996. You'll find this book, written by a mother and physician, interesting and helpful. It's for parents of children with ADHD who are looking for answers other than medication.

Conners, C. K. *Feeding the Brain: How Foods Affect Children*. New York: Plenum Press, 1989. Dr. Conners is well respected nationally for his work with hyperactive children. This interesting book explores the links between diet and behavior.

Crook, W. G. *Help for the Hyperactive Child*. Jackson, TN: Professional Books, 1997. Since the 1950s Dr. Crook has been helping children with behavior and health problems by identifying problem foods in their diets and chemicals in their environment. You'll find this book a practical guide for parents of children with ADHD who are looking for alternatives to Ritalin.

Crook, W. G. *Tracking Down Hidden Food Allergy*. Jackson, TN: Professional Books, 1995. If you suspect your child has food sensitivities, this book will help you track down which foods bother your child. Its easy-to-read style will lead you through elimination diets with suggested menus and recipes.

Crook, W. G. *The Yeast Connection Handbook*. Jackson, TN: Professional Books, 2000. If your child has had repeated ear infections and many antibiotics, this book is an excellent guide for understanding and overcoming yeast-related behavior and health problems.

Crook, W. G., and L. J. Stevens. *Solving the Puzzle of Your Hard-to-Raise Child*. New York: Random House, 1987. Dr. Crook and I teamed up to write this book to help parents solve the puzzling problems of their children who had behavior, health, and learning problems.

Galland, L. *The Four Pillars of Healing*. New York: Random House, 1997. Although this book doesn't specifically address the problems of children with ADHD, you will find Dr. Galland's approach to alternative and traditional treatments exciting and enlightening.

Galland, L. *Superimmunity for Kids*. New York: Copestone Press, 1988. This outstanding guide will help you feed your child healthy foods so he can enjoy optimal health. It also discusses what supplements your child should take.

Hersey, J. *Why Can't My Child Behave?* Alexandria, VA: Pear Tree Press, 1996. This book is an excellent guide to the Feingold Diet, which was popular in the 1970s and continues to help children today.

Irlen, H. *Reading by the Colors*. Garden City Park, NY: Avery Publishing Group, 1991. This is the first book to explain the Irlen method of reading with colored lenses, a method that has helped many children improve reading skills.

O'Dell, N. E., and P. A. Cook. *Stopping Hyperactivity: A New Solution*. Garden City Park, NY: Avery Publishing Group, 1997. These professors of education at the University of Indianapolis have developed a new way to help hyperactive children with a unique exercise program.

Rapp, D. J. *The Impossible Child*. Tacoma, WA: Life Sciences Press, 1986. This book, by a ground-breaking pediatrician, is a helpful guide for teachers and parents who are trying to figure out why a child is inattentive, impulsive, and overactive at school and at home.

Sears, W., and L. Thompson. *The A.D.D. Book*. New York: Little, Brown, 1998. This is an outstanding book with lots of helpful information. It will answer many of your questions about diagnosis, behavior modification, learning problems, biofeedback, and diet.

Truss, C. O. *The Missing Diagnosis*. Birmingham, AL, 1985 (available from PO Box 26508, Birmingham AL 35226). Dr. Truss is a pioneer in connecting problems with yeast with behavior and health problems.

Internet Resources

The ADD/ADHD Online Newsletter
Web address: http://www.nlci.com

This is my own home page, which has news for parents, questions and comments from readers, recipes, references from the medical literature for you and your doctor, and links to other helpful websites. Each month the topics change. Tune in and I'll keep you abreast of what's new in research and treatment for ADD and ADHD.

Asthma and Allergy Foundation of America
Web address: http://pslgroup.com/dg/6d0a.htm

The Asthma and Allergy Foundation of America provides tips for parents to reduce exposure to airborne allergens and other helpful information for parents of allergic children.

Sidney M. Baker, M.D.

Web address: http://www.sbakermd.com

Dr. Sidney Baker has been helping children and adults with chronic behavior and health problems for many years. He has been successful in treating patients who have failed with other doctors' treatment. On his website Dr. Baker shares his vast knowledge of and experience regarding food allergies, magnesium, yeast, and more.

Candida-Yeast Website

Web address: http://www.candida-yeast.com

This website is the creation of William G. Crook, M.D., who has worked for decades to assist children and adults with food sensitivities and a yeast problem. If you suspect your child may have a problem with the common yeast *Candida albicans*, consult this site for plenty of useful information.

Center for Science in the Public Interest (CSPI)

Web address: http://www.cspinet.org/

This national organization is at the forefront of fighting for the health of consumers concerned about nutrition. You'll like their home page. They have many topics you can explore. They also publish a monthly newsletter, "Nutrition Action," that will keep you abreast of all the latest nutrition concerns.

Diet, ADHD, and Behavior is an exciting new booklet published by CSPI. If your doctor or psychologist is skeptical about the role of foods and additives in ADHD, this booklet is ideal. It summarizes and cites all the studies that have explored a link between food sensitivities and ADD/ADHD. It will not only help your doctor to help your child, but it will help her help other children, too. You can order it by sending a check or money order for $8.00 to: CSPI, 1875 Connecticut Avenue, NW, Suite 300, Washington, DC 20009-5728. CSPI also publishes a helpful pamphlet for parents for $1.50. These booklets will change a lot of minds—and a lot of lives.

Children and Adults with Attention Deficit Disorder (CHADD)
Web address: http://www.chadd.org/

This national support group is dedicated to bringing you accurate, current information on medical, scientific, educational, and advocacy issues. It sponsors conferences and offers a newsletter, *Attention.* This group supports the use of medication and was chastised recently because it had received money from the makers of Ritalin. CHADD does not support the idea that diet has anything to do with behavior. Nevertheless, it has many local support groups where parents can discuss their problems with other parents who understand.

CNN Allergy Report
Web address: http://cnn.com/WEATHER/allergy/

This is a great web page if you're interested in finding out grass, tree, and weed pollen and mold levels in your geographic area. This may help you make some connection between your child's behavior and health symptoms and these common allergens.

Feingold Association of the United States
Web address: http://www.feingold.org/index.html

This national organization has been working since the 1970s to help children with ADHD modify their diets by eliminating artificial colors and flavors, preservatives, and natural foods containing aspirin-like chemicals (salicylates). This is the diet that was promoted by pediatric allergist Benjamin Feingold, M.D., in the early 1970s. When you become a member of the Feingold Association you will receive all kinds of helpful information. The association publishes an interesting newsletter, *The Pure Facts.*

Foundation for Integrated Medicine
Web address: http://www.mdheal.org

This website is sponsored by Leo Galland, M.D., and the Foundation for Integrated Medicine. Integrated medicine draws on the best treatments available whether they are in alternative care or traditional medicine. The foundation is especially interested in the health of children. You'll like this site.

Human Ecology Action League (HEAL)
Web address: http://member.aol.com/HEALNatnl/index.html

HEAL is a nonprofit foundation that for the last twenty-three years has provided information and education about the effects of environmental and chemical exposures from the perspective of noted professionals, as well as from those who have experienced and dealt with numerous exposure-related illnesses including ADD/ADHD. The foundation publishes an excellent quarterly newsletter, *The Human Ecologist*. You can contact HEAL at PO Box 29629, Atlanta GA 30359-0629.

Hyperactive Children's Support Group
Web address: http://www.geocities.com/HotSprings/2125/

This organization in the United Kingdom is for patients with ADD/ADHD, parents of hyperactive children, and professionals. This group does not advocate the use of drugs as a treatment for hyperactivity. Instead, it helps parents try dietary modifications.

Parents of Allergic Children (PAC)
Web address: http://drone.simplenet.com/pac/

PAC provides support and information to parents whose children suffer from allergies to foods, chemicals, and the environment. PAC is particularly interested in children with learning or behavioral problems due to allergies and nutrition. PAC publishes *Allergic Times Newsletter*.

Pub Med (National Library of Medicine)
Web address: http://www.ncbi.nlm.nih.gov/PubMed

This website is a treasure. You can easily search 9 million scientific medical references in a few minutes by typing in your search terms. Type in "ADHD fatty acids," for example, and you'll get all the references that deal with ADHD and fatty acids. You can then print out the abstracts of interesting articles. If you want to know still more, you can ask your librarian to order these publications for you on Interlibrary Loan. Knowledge is power and this website gives you the latest scientific research.

Newsgroups

You can subscribe to these two newsgroups, to ask questions and receive answers from other parents and adults struggling with ADD and ADHD:

alt.support.attn-deficit

alt.parenting.solutions

Conferences

"Attention Deficit Hyperactivity Disorder: Causes and Possible Solutions"

This conference, held November 4–7, 1999, in Arlington, Virginia, was sponsored by the prestigious Georgetown University Medical Center and the International Health Foundation. Program participants discussed a variety of topics dealing with conventional and nonconventional approaches to the diagnosis and treatment of ADHD and other related disorders. The syllabus, of more than 200 pages, is available for $25 from: International Health Foundation, 45 Conrad Drive, Jackson, TN 38305. Audiotapes are available from: Insta Tapes, PO Box 908, Coeur d'Alene, ID 83316; telephone 1-208-667-0226.

NOTES

What Are ADD and ADHD?

1. American Psychiatric Association, *Diagnostic and Statistical Manual of Mental Disorders (DSM-IV)* (Washington, DC: APA, 1994).
2. R. A. Barkley, *Attention-Deficit Hyperactivity Disorder: A Handbook for Diagnosis and Treatment* (New York: Guilford Press, 1998), 97–126.
3. Ibid., 99.
4. Ibid., 122.
5. Ibid., 37–38.
6. W. G. Crook and L. J. Stevens, *Solving the Puzzle of Your Hard-to-Raise Child* (New York: Random House and Professional Books, 1987), 79.
7. R. B. Kanarek and R. Marks-Kaufman, *Nutrition and Behavior* (New York: Van Nostrand Reinhold, 1991).
8. P. Hauser et al., "Attention-Deficit-Hyperactivity Disorder in People with Generalized Resistance to Thyroid Hormone," *New England*

Journal of Medicine 328 (1993): 997–1001; R. Weiss et al., "Attention-Deficit Hyperactivity Disorder and Thyroid Function," *Journal of Pediatrics* 123 (1993): 539–45. Letters to the Editor, "ADHD and the Thyroid," *Journal of the Academy of Child and Adolescent Psychiatry* 33 (1994): 1057–58.

9. R. Weiss, "Behavioral Effects of Liothyronine (L-T3) in Children with Attention Deficit Hyperactivity Disorder in the Presence and Absence of Resistance to Thyroid Hormone," *Thyroid* 7 (1997): 389–93.

10. M. A. Block, *No More Ritalin* (New York: Kensington Books, 1996), 48–49.

11. Barkley, *Attention-Deficit Hyperactivity Disorder*, 568–69.

12. C. W. Popper, "Combining Methylphenidate and Clonidine," *Journal of Child and Adolescent Psychopharmacy* 5 (1995): 157–66.

13. Barkley, *Attention-Deficit Hyperactivity Disorder*, 568.

14. *Physicians' Desk Reference* (Montvale, NJ: Medical Economics, 1998), 1897.

15. J. M. Swanson, "Effect of Stimulant Medication on Children with Attention Deficit Disorder: A Review of Reviews," *Exceptional Children* 60 (1993): 154–62.

Causes of ADD and ADHD

1. Barkley, *Attention-Deficit Hyperactivity Disorder*, 170–73.

An Ounce of Prevention

1. G. M. Wardlaw and P. M. Insel, *Perspectives in Nutrition* (St. Louis: Mosby, 1996), 595.

2. A. Lucas et al., "Breast Milk and Subsequent Intelligence Quotient in Children Born Preterm," *Lancet* 339 (1992): 261–64.

3. Allergy Information Association Newsletter, "Feeding a Baby with Allergies" (March 1972): 1–2.

Way 1. Improve Your Child's Diet

1. Crook and Stevens, *Solving the Puzzle of Your Hard-to-Raise Child*, 5, 30; L. Galland, *Superimmunity for Kids* (New York: Copestone Press, 1988), 12, 142–44.

2. K. A. Munoz, "Food Intakes of U.S. Children and Adolescents Compared with Recommendation," *Pediatrics* 100 (1997): 323–29.

3. Ibid.

4. L. Cornelius, "Health Habits of School-Age Children," *Journal of Health Care for the Poor and Underserved* 2 (1991): 374–95.

5. J. M. Murphy, "The Relationship of School Breakfast to Psychosocial and Academic Functioning," *Archives of Pediatric and Adolescent Medicine* 152 (1998): 899–907.

6. W. Sears and L. Thompson, *The A.D.D. Book* (New York: Little, Brown, 1994), 271.

7. Crook, *Help for the Hyperactive Child*, 214–15.

8. Crook and Stevens, *Solving the Puzzle of Your Hard-to-Raise Child*, 182.

Way 2. Choose Sweeteners Carefully

1. H. E. Wender and M. V. Solanto, "Effects of Sugar on Aggressive and Inattentive Behavior in Children with Attention Deficit Disorder with Hyperactivity and Normal Children," *Pediatrics* 88 (1991): 960–66; R. J. Prinz, "Dietary Correlates of Hyperactive Behavior in Children," *Journal of Consulting Clinical Psychology* 48 (1980): 760–69; J. A. Goldman, "Behavioral Effects of Sucrose on Preschool Children," *Journal of Abnormal Child Psychology* 14 (1986): 565 77; J. Egger et al., "Controlled Trial of Oligoantigenic Treatment in the Hyperkinetic Syndrome," *Lancet* 1 (1985): 540–45; M. L. Wolraich et al., "Effects of Diets High in Sucrose or Aspartame on the Behavior and Cognitive Performance of Children," *New England Journal of Medicine* 330 (1994): 301–307; M. L.Wolraich, "The Effect of Sugar on Behavior or Cognition in Children," *Journal of the American Medical Association* 274 (1995): 1617–12; D. Behar et al., "Sugar Challenge Testing with Children Considered Behaviorally Sugar Reactive," *Nutrition and Behavior* 1 (1984): 277–88; R. Milich and W. E. Pelham, "The Effects of Sugar on the Classroom and Playgroup Behavior of Attention Deficit Disordered Boys," *Journal of Consulting and Clinical Psychology* 54 (1986): 1–5.

2. S. J. Schoenthaler, "Sugar and Children's Behavior," *New England Journal of Medicine* 350 (1994): 1901.

3. C. K. Conners, *Feeding the Brain* (New York: Plenum Press, 1989), 25–47.

4. Wolraich et al., "Effects of Diets," 301–307.

Way 4. Add Essential Fatty Acids

1. A. Venuta et al., "Essential Fatty Acids: the Effects of Dietary Supplementation Among Children with Recurrent Respiratory Infections," *Journal of International Medical Research* (1996): 325–30.

2. E. A. Mitchell et al., "Clinical Characteristics and Serum Essential Fatty Acid Levels in Hyperactive Children," *Clinical Pediatrics* 26 (1987): 406–11.

3. M. Neuringer et al., "The Essentiality of N-3 Fatty Acids for the Development and Function of the Retina and Brain," *Annual Review of Nutrition* 8 (1988): 517–41; S. Reisbick et al., "Polydipsia in Rhesus Monkeys Deficient in Omega-3 Fatty Acids," *Physiology and Behavior* 47 (1990): 315–23; S. Reisbick et al., "Home Cage Behavior of Rhesus Monkeys with Long-Term Deficiency of Omega-3 Fatty Acids," *Physiology and Behavior* 55 (1994): 231–39.

Way 5. Choose Vitamins, Minerals, and Other Supplements Carefully

1. S. J. Shoenthaler et al., "The Effect of Vitamin-Mineral Supplementation on Juvenile Delinquency Among American Schoolchildren: A Randomized Double-Blind Placebo-Controlled Trial," *Journal of Alternative and Complementary Medicine: Research on Paradigm, Practice, and Policy* 6 (2000): 19–29; S. J Shoenthaler et al., "Controlled Trial of Vitamin-Mineral Supplementation on Intelligence and Brain Function," *Personality and Individual Difference* 112 (1991): 343–50.

2. Galland, *Superimmunity for Kids*, 180.

3. A. Brenner, "The Effects of Megadoses of Selected B Complex Vitamins on Children with Hyperkinesis: Controlled Studies with Long-Term Follow-up," *Journal of Learning Disabilities* 15 (1982): 258–64.

4. J. Z. Miller et al., "Therapeutic Effect of Vitamin C: A Co-Twin Controlled Study," *Journal of the American Medical Association* 237 (1977): 248–51.

5. T. Kozielec et al., "Deficiency of Certain Trace Elements in Children with Hyperactivity," *Psychiatria Polska* 28 (1994): 345–53.

6. T. Kozielec and B. Starobrat-Hermelin, "Assessment of Magnesium Levels in Children with ADHD," *Magnesium Research* 10 (1997): 143–48; B. Starobrat-Hermelin and T. Kozielec, "The Effects of Magnesium Physiological Supplementation on Hyperactivity in Children with ADHD: Positive Response to Magnesium Oral Loading Test," *Magnesium Research* 10 (1997): 149–56.

7. L. Galland, "Magnesium and the Battle for Light," *Gesell Institute of Human Development Update* 4 (1985): 4–5.

8. Galland, *Superimmunity for Kids*, 137.

9. P. Toren et al., "Zinc Deficiency in Attention Deficit Hyperactivity Disorder," *Biological Psychiatry* 40 (1996): 1308–10.

10. Galland, *Superimmunity for Kids*, 161.

11. S. B. Mossad et al., "Zinc Gluconate Lozenges for Treating the Common Cold: A Randomized, Double-Blind, Placebo-Controlled Study," *Annals of Internal Medicine* 125 (1996): 81–83.

12. L. Michael et al., "Zinc Gluconate Lozenges for Treating the Common Cold in Children," *Journal of the American Medical Association* 279 (1996): 1962–67.

13. K. D. Dwykman and R. A. Dwykman, "Effect of Nutritional Supplements on Attention-Deficit Hyperactivity Disorder," *Integrative Physiological and Behavioral Science* 33 (1998): 49–60; K. D. Dwykman and R. A. Dwykman, "Effect of Glyconutrients on the Severity of ADHD," *Proceedings of the Fisher Institute for Medical Research* 1 (1997): 24–25.

14. H. Zhang and J. Huang, "Preliminary Study of Traditional Chinese Medicine Treatment of Minimal Brain Dysfunction," *Chung Hsi I Chieh Ho Tsa Chih Chinese Journal of Modern Developments in Traditional Medicine* 10 (1990): 278–79.

15. L. H. Wang et al. "Clinical and Experimental Studies on Tiaoshen Liquor for Infantile Hyperkinetic Syndrome," *Chung-Kuo Chung Hsi I Chieh Ho Tsa Chih* 15 (1995): 337–40.

Way 6. Solve the Yeast Connection

1. C. O. Truss, *The Missing Diagnosis* (Birmingham, AL: Missing Diagnosis, 1985).
2. Ibid., 71, 90.
3. K. Iwata, "Toxins Reproduced by *Candida albicans*," *Contributions in Microbiology and Immunology* 4 (1977): 77–85.
4. Galland, *Superimmunity for Kids*, 171.
5. Gesell Institute, *Basic Elements—News* 1 (1986): 1–4.
6. Crook and Stevens, *Solving the Puzzle of Your Hard-to-Raise Child*, 145–48.
7. W. G. Crook, *The Yeast Connection Handbook* (Jackson, TN: Professional Books, 2000), 128–34.

Way 7. Identify Inhalant Allergies

1. F. Simons, "Learning Impairment and Allergic Rhinitis," *Allergy and Asthma Proceedings* 17 (1996): 185–89.

Way 9. Investigate Lead and Aluminum Poisoning

1. Conversation with Sidney Baker, M.D., 2000.
2. F. L. Ilg, L. B. Ames, and S. M. Baker, *Child Behavior* (New York: Harper & Row, 1981), 303.

Way 10. Enhance Perception

1. H. Irlen, *Reading by the Colors* (Garden City Park, NY: Avery Publishing Group, 1991), 43.
2. Quoted ibid., 13–14.
3. Quoted ibid., 19.
4. P. D. O'Connor et al., "Reading Disabilities and the Effects of Colored Filters," *Journal of Learning Disabilities* 23 (1990): 597–620.
5. G. L. Robinson, P. J. Foreman, and K. B. Dear, "The Familial Incidence of Symptoms of Scotopic Sensitivity Syndrome," *Perceptual and Motor Skills* 83 (1996): 1043–55; G. L. Robinson and R. N. Conway, "Irlen Filters and Reading Strategies: Effect of Coloured Filters on Reading Achievement, Specific Reading Strategies, and Perception of

Ability," *Perceptual and Motor Skills* 79 (1994): 467–83; C. Sawyer and S. Taylor, "Transparent Coloured Overlays and Specific Learning Disabilities," *Educational Psychology in Practice* 9 (1994): 217–20; O'Connor et al., "Reading Disabilities," 597–620.

6. Irlen, *Reading by the Colors*, 74.
7. M. S. Kreuttnew and I. Strum, "The Irlen Approach: An Intervention for Students with Low Reading Achievement and Symptoms of Scotopic Sensitivity Syndrome," 1990.
8. K. Owre and L. Bryant, "Innovations in Reading Programming for LD Students." Report for the Las Cruces, New Mexico, Public Schools.
9. Personal communication with Irlen, 1999.
10. Ibid.
11. J. N. Ott, *Light, Radiation and You* (Old Greenwich, CT: Devon-Adair, 1982), 130–33.
12. Personal communication with Irlen, 1999.

Way 11. Consider Crawling Lessons
1. N. E. O'Dell and P. A. Cook, *Stopping Hyperactivity: A New Solution* (Garden City Park, NY: Avery Publishing Group, 1997), 8.
2. Ibid., 69.
3. Ibid., 9.
4. Personal communication with O'Dell and Cook, 1999.
5. O'Dell and Cook, *Stopping Hyperactivity*, 43–44.
6. M. L. Bender, "A Study of the Relationship Between Persistent Immaturity of the Symmetric Tonic Neck Reflex and Learning Disabilities in Children," Ph.D. dissertation, Purdue University, 1971.
7. N. A. O'Dell, "Study of the Relationship of Bender Resisted Exercises to the Symmetric Tonic Neck Reflex and to Achievement Test Scores," Ph.D. dissertation, Purdue University, 1973.

Way 12. Try Biofeedback
1. J. F. Lubar et al., "Evaluation of the Effectiveness of EEG Neurofeedback Training for ADHD in a Clinical Setting as Measured by

Changes in T.O.V.A. Scores, Behavioral Ratings, and WISC-R Performance," *Biofeedback and Self-Regulation* 20 (1995): 83–89.

2. J. F. Lubar, "Neurofeedback for the Management of Attention-Deficit /Hyperactivity Disorders," in Mark Schwartz, ed., *Biofeedback: A Practitioner's Guide* (New York: Guilford Press, 1995), 493.

3. M. A. Tansey and R. L. Bruner, "EMG and EEG Biofeedback Training in the Treatment of a 10-Year-Old Hyperactive Boy with a Developmental Reading Disorder," *Biofeedback and Self-Regulation* 8 (1983): 25–37.

4. Ibid.

5. D. B. Kotwal et al., "Computer-Assisted Cognitive Training for ADHD: A Case Study," *Behavior Modification* 20 (1996): 85–97.

6. Ibid.

7. W. Sears and L. Thompson, *The A.D.D. Book* (Boston: Little, Brown, 1998), 217.

8. Lubar et al., "Evaluation of the Effectiveness of EEG Neurofeedback Training."

9. Ibid., 99.

10. T. R. Rossiter and T. J. La Vaque, "A Comparison of EEG Biofeedback and Psychostimulants in Treating Attention Deficit/Hyperactivity Disorders," *Journal of Neurotherapy* (1995): 48–59.

11. Ibid., 57.

12. Sears and Thompson, *The A.D.D. Book*, 224.

Conclusion

1. L. Galland, Letters to the Editor, *U.S. News & World Report* (Nov. 7, 1998).

2. L. E. Arnold, "Treatment Alternatives for Attention-Deficit Hyperactivity Disorder (ADHD)," *Journal of Attention Disorders* 3 (1999): 30–48.

3. Conners, *Feeding the Brain*, 255.

INDEX

ABOUT THE AUTHOR

For more than twenty-five years, Laura Stevens has been researching the role of nutrition and food sensitivities in ADD/ADHD, and she is considered a pioneer in this important field of study. She received her master of science degree in food and nutrition from Purdue University. In addition to her practice as a nutritional counselor, Stevens gives frequent lectures on ADD/ADHD and is currently working on a study at Purdue on the effects of essential fatty acid supplementation and ADHD. Founder and president of Nutrition in Action, Inc., the developer of *The ADD/ADHD Online Newsletter* (www.nlci.com/nutrition), and a coauthor of *How to Feed Your Hyperactive Child,* among several other books, she lives in Lafayette, Indiana, with her husband.